Contents

Acknowledgements iv

Introduction v

Part one: Communication barriers 1

one Process barriers 3

two Structural barriers 15

Part two: Intervention studies 31

three Intervention studies: service development 33

four Intervention studies: advocates and linkworkers 51

five Intervention studies: interpreters 73

six Intervention studies: training 93

seven Intervention studies: health education programmes and resources 125

eight Conclusions 157

References 167

Appendix 1: Protocol extracts 181

Appendix 2: Data extraction form 185

Appendix 3: Search strategies example: PsychLIT 193

Appendix 4: Tables 195

Index 201

Acknowledgements

I owe a considerable debt to various collaborators who have offered generous encouragement and made it possible for this report to be written. The Steering Group of the Overcoming Barriers and Enhancing Communication (OBEC) project at the School of Healthcare Studies, University of Leeds, encouraged the drafting of this text as part of a larger project, funded by the School, which has been investigating strategies for overcoming barriers and enhancing communication between health service providers and service users who are not fluent in English. The members of the project Steering Group are Jo Green, Peter Knapp, Janet Hirst, Kuldip Bharj, Joe Cortis, Shupi Rinomhota, Jo Gilmartin and Pauline Phillips, and I wish to acknowledge and thank them for all their comments, advice and support. I particularly thank Jo Green for her valuable comments on the draft typescript. Janet Hirst made useful suggestions concerning the 'communication' section in the Introduction. Jo Gilmartin also made an important contribution in significantly helping with redrafting the communication barriers material. In addition, Fiona Van Marken, also of the School of Healthcare Studies, helped substantially with the collection of research papers, the implementation of the review process using a pre-screen form and a data extraction form, and with critical comments on drafts. Ian Law of the University of Leeds Department of Sociology and Centre for Ethnicity and Racism Studies provided helpful comments on the sections on ethnicity and racism. The literature search strategies were developed with the guidance of Janette Boynton at the Health Sciences Library, University of Leeds. Thanks also to Aliya Darr (Centre for Research in Primary Care, Leeds) and Nancy Lester (Leeds Teaching Hospitals NHS Trust) for their support.

Introduction

Background and context of research

This book examines existing research into communication between health care providers and minority ethnic[1] health care users who lack fluency[2] in English. The book should be of value to academics, researchers, and students in health care and also the sociology of health, and to health service practitioners and leaders. It takes account of research conducted within health care disciplines, while complementing this with perspectives derived from the sociology of health and communication. The strong dual focus on empirical research and on communication sets it apart from other books focused on minority ethnic users and health, which have tended to have a less empirical flavour (Robinson, 1998), or to focus more generally on ethnicity (Ahmad, 1993).

The book does not exhaustively explore the full range of barriers to health care facing minority ethnic patients. Many members of minority ethnic groups in the UK do not lack fluency in English; an increasing number are born and raised here. Yet many of the communication barriers they face doubtless overlap with those of non-fluent speakers, for example concerning institutional and attitudinal rather than strictly linguistic factors; however, not all the research touching on their needs is covered here. At the same time, the scope of the book remains wide-ranging, and it includes research conducted in several countries where English is a national language, widely used in health care, particularly the US, Canada, and Australia, as well as the UK. As a result, a considerable diversity of minority ethnic groups and health care contexts is considered. Some facets of the research are rather context-dependent, indeed the robustness of communication research may require context-sensitivity, yet many aspects of each study should have broad application wherever minority ethnic users not fluent in English strive to have their communication needs understood and met. Given that the number of interventions in this area remains small, a strength of this study should be the broad scope it offers for making careful comparisons.

The primary focus is on empirical evidence of barriers to

communication, and of interventions aimed at enhancing communication, involving minority service users who are less than fluent in English. However, the book cannot consider all minority ethnic community groups in English-speaking countries, since relevant interventions have not been carried out involving many such minorities. A substantial amount of research in the UK has focused on South Asian minority ethnic communities, whereas the needs of others, such as Polish, Vietnamese; and new migrants, including asylum seekers, are as yet relatively under-researched. User groups with particularly complex needs and affiliations such as minority ethnic people with disabilities, and older people also seem relatively under-represented. Men's concerns may also receive less attention than women's concerns in the pages that follow.

What is not in doubt is that for many members of under-represented groups, including new migrants whose importance for the health service is bound to increase, issues of communication are central. Lack of fluency in English is one of the most significant among several interacting factors influencing the health care experiences of these service users and an understanding of the current evidence, with its strengths and also its weaknesses, is likely to be of increasing importance to health service practitioners and academics.

During a period of major reforms, the health service in Britain has been subject to important debates about accountability and accessibility to users. UK government policy documents have supported action to address the needs of minority ethnic users. For example, the government White Paper *Saving lives: Our healthier nation* (DoH, 1999a) set a framework and provided an action plan for health improvements, especially for the "worst off" (p 1, para 1.2) which carries implications for communication needs. The Department of Health (DoH) circular *Clinical governance* (DoH, 1999b) explicitly linked an agenda for continuing professional development with reducing health inequalities and targeting minority ethnic service users and carers. The document *The vital connection: An equalities framework for the NHS* (DoH, 2000) emphasises setting and maintaining equality standards and prioritises promotion of education to meet the needs of culturally diverse communities. The document *Making a difference* (DoH, 1999c) set out a "new vision" (p 6) for nurses, midwives and health visitors in the NHS, explicitly requiring these practitioners to target the most vulnerable in the community, including some minority ethnic groups, who are least likely to access and use the service.

Rhetorical recognition of the importance of cultural and ethnic diversity to the delivery of an equitable service does not mean that the health service and health practitioners meet the needs of minority ethnic patients effectively (M. Johnson, 1996). Recognising and meeting the needs of all service users depends on structures and processes of communication. In fact, relationships between understanding needs, service development, and communication processes, are often mutually informing and require conceptual and empirical attention. In that general context a number of issues, linked to communication, concern non-fluent minority ethnic health care users specifically. The main body of this book examines the evidence concerning these issues and explores implications for practice and for policy.

Issues, where evidence is available concerning non-fluent service users, relate to:

- equal opportunities for access and participation for service users who may not be fluent in English, among diverse client groups;
- organisational constraints on the provision of communication support in the health service;
- unease about institutional racism;
- attitudes and practices of some health care professionals;
- concerns about the use of material resources.

A first concern is that a service which aims to provide equal opportunities for health for all requires equitable processes supporting access and participation for diverse and marginalised client groups. A further problem, as later chapters show, is that structural and organisational constraints in the health service disadvantage users who lack fluency in English. The constraints include the quality of mechanisms for planning, implementing and monitoring ethnically sensitive service development (Monach and Davis, 1996).

Another issue is that health service reforms are occurring in a period of increasing awareness of institutional racism and concern to understand and challenge the mechanisms which support it. The MacPherson Report (1999) defines institutional racism in terms of the systematic differential treatment of people by organisations because of their race, and emphasises that the definition rests on the effects of organisational practice, and not intentions. With the 2000 Race Relations (Amendment) Act public authorities in the UK now have a strengthened statutory duty to examine discriminatory practices and promote racial equality. Discriminatory practice can happen in any kind of care work, but it becomes particularly possible where language barriers exist, and when health professionals are stretched to their limits.

Also, a related and enduring concern is that the attitudes and practices of some health professionals to minority ethnic service users remain unacceptable (Rocheron et al, 1989; Murphy and Macleod Clark, 1993). Stereotyping or over-controlling behaviour, in relation to assumptions about cultural difference and language deficit, may contribute to instances of two-way miscommunication, and a reluctance to request or use appropriate language support resources (Gerrish, 2001). A further problem is that the provision of material resources to meet the education or information needs of minority ethnic service users is woefully inadequate in many places. There are not enough appropriately translated materials and not enough materials in appropriate media, for example visually formatted (Arora et al, 1995; Karim, 1996).

The book highlights these concerns by assessing the available evidence. At the same time, gaps in the research are discussed. The majority of interventions under-emphasise the contexts of communications between service users and providers. Too little is known about the socio-cultural environments within which people's needs are felt and expressed, and which influence the effectiveness of communications. The diversity of sub-cultures is flattened out in interventions, so that, for example, the focus on minority ethnic women and health is not often matched by a sharp interest in socio-economic differentials, nor by a focus on such specific groups as people with disabilities, nor, indeed, on men. Equally there is a need to understand better the specific and dynamic work contexts where practitioners' perceptions occur as they communicate.

Addressing such a range of issues is a central challenge for health providers. The variable quality and limited quantity of relevant empirical research aimed at enhancing communication perhaps reflects the continued marginalisation of minority ethnic service users' concerns. This book therefore sets out to be both descriptive and evaluative, and to offer a useful guide to the evidence for practitioners, health educators, researchers in the field, students, service users and service managers.

Aims

The primary aim of this book is to evaluate the research evidence relating to communication between adult minority ethnic service users who lack fluency in English and health care professionals, so as to inform practice and service development, and to identify the most pressing research issues. A large, central section of the book focuses on reviewing empirical studies that have aimed to enhance health communications with minority ethnic clients who lack fluency in English. Earlier sections more briefly identify barriers to effective communication. Empirical studies of barriers are reviewed in a wide range of areas, including those of consultation and needs assessment for service development, health professionals' communication practice, bilingual services, health education programmes and materials, service organisation and management, and training of health professionals. The Introduction also highlights important conceptual issues for research in key areas concerning ethnicity, racism, culture and communication. The effectiveness of actions taken to enhance communication depends in part on whether the issues have been adequately conceptualised for operational research or for service development. It also depends in part on whether barriers which have been identified are adequately confronted through the interventions. A central argument of the book, in fact, is that overcoming barriers and enhancing communication with minority ethnic service users requires the development of an adequate conceptual and empirical toolkit for understanding the issues and tackling them.

Methods

Advisory panel

A panel of advisors contributed to the planning of the review and provided feedback on the focus and direction.

Study protocol

A study protocol or structured plan was developed with a set of objectives for the review and specific criteria for the selection of papers for review. The set of objectives is shown in Appendix I.

The objectives were met by a review of healthcare literature which includes:

- a summary review of conceptual frameworks relevant to the research;
- a summary evaluative review of empirical 'barrier' studies;
- a structured review of interventions.

The review of interventions both describes the range of interventions that have been carried out, and evaluates their quality. The conceptual review provides an underpinning for evaluation of the way key concepts are used operationally, and how this affects the validity of the research. The barriers review underpins evaluation of how adequately the interventions address the range of major barriers to communication.

Selection of studies for the review

The conceptual review includes some work from health care, sociology and linguistics. Interdisciplinary work is emphasised since health service research and development has been influenced by specific conceptual frameworks indebted to other disciplinary fields.

A set of necessary criteria, shown in Appendix 1, was devised to select the empirical studies for review. For reasons of feasibility, studies eligible for inclusion in the electronic database search dated from January 1989 to March 2000, English language only. However, where the studies in the review cite earlier studies of central importance, these were also considered. Some background research published since that date is also included.

Search strategy

A search strategy was developed with the assistance of the advisory panel and of librarians at the University of Leeds. Both electronic and hand searches were carried out. Search terms and a list of databases used are shown in Appendix 1, and a sample search in Appendix 3.

Results of the literature search

Papers identified

As a result of a pre-screening process a total of 25 interventions, 62 empirical barrier studies, and 47 concept studies were collected for review.

Development of data extraction form

A data extraction form was developed to collect descriptive and evaluative information about the intervention studies. Headings are shown in Appendix 2.

Some of the criteria for evaluating qualitative, interpretative research differ from criteria for evaluating quantitative, positivist research, despite specific challenges for the evaluation of 'hybrid' studies using multi-method designs.

The healthcare field abounds with material on developing criteria for quantitative research. However, many quantitative studies have paid relatively little attention to service user perspectives, and provide little information about processes and contexts. They are then not always suitable for addressing a range of health communication issues that are multi-dimensional, and concern subjective or inter-subjective meanings. On the other hand, it has been argued that good qualitative research attends to the interpretation of subjective meaning and the adequate description of social contexts, and that in such cases adequacy needs to be assessed at the level of meanings which can help to explain why something happens or is the way that it is (Popay et al, 1998). Therefore, criteria for the evaluation of qualitative research were developed, drawing on existing theoretical and empirical work (Mays and Pope, 1995; Lemmer et al, 1999; Newman, 1999). These criteria are applied in relevant parts of this book.

Presentation of review findings

All selected research studies were reviewed. A brief review of key conceptual issues precedes a summary review of barriers to communication, and then the detailed review of interventions.

The review of barriers focuses on the following central issues, identified from the empirical studies:

* stereotyping
* language and miscommunication
* the adaptation of prevailing practice models to transcultural communication contexts
* assessment of minority ethnic user needs by community consultation
* gathering and use of information about individual patients' communication needs

- bilingual support
- practitioner education
- provision of material resources.

The review of the intervention studies includes the following areas:

- evaluation of service organisation
- ethnic matching, and service matching
- ethnic monitoring
- bilingual services – advocates, linkworkers and interpreters
- training – health care professionals and staff
- training interpreters and implementing an interpreter service
- health education programmes
- material resources and media.

Issues arising from the study

The concluding section highlights key findings and focuses on the implications of the study for research, for evidence-based practice, and for health service development. It emphasises what has been achieved, and what remains to be achieved in understanding and acting on urgent issues for enhancing communication between health service providers and minority ethnic service users who are not fluent in English.

Conceptual issues

In any empirical research inconsistent and confusing operational use of the concepts leads to flawed interventions. The process of conceptual clarification can therefore be helpful for evaluating research and development in health care settings. The brief summary here of current debates on ethnicity, racism, culture and communication is intended to inform the subsequent review of empirical research on communication involving minority ethnic health service users who are not fluent speakers of English.

Ethnicity

Definitions of ethnicity

Definitions of ethnicity in health research are problematic – for example, the words culture and ethnicity are not always clearly distinguished when used together. The concept of ethnicity is fiercely debated (Annandale, 1999). A review of the theoretical literature on ethnicity suggest two persistent tendencies – to define ethnicity in 'primordial' terms and in 'instrumental' ones (Smaje, 1996, p 141). Both tendencies view ethnicity, with varying emphasis, in terms of boundaries and continuities. The former views ethnicity as, in the last resort, a social construct by which people gain a fundamental orientation to the world (in the sense of 'ethnic identity'). The latter views ethnicity as a social construct instrumental for accessing resources (Smaje, 1996, p 141). Operational definitions may also relate ethnicity to a cluster of other concepts that supply criteria for the differentiation of social groups. The criteria may include: language (viewed as a distinct language or as a distinct dialect), common origin (or 'homeland' from which the group migrated), common religion, common history and culture (Law, 1996, pp 43-4).

Significant developments in the theorisation of ethnicity include structural-materialist views of competing material interests of social classes impacting on definitions of ethnicity (Smaje, 1996, p 145). Alternatively, with the notion of situational ethnicity, individuals can adopt ethnic labels in different contexts for different purposes (Smaje, 1996, p 141). There is considerable interest from situational and post-modern perspectives in how ethnicities are produced and reproduced, defined and redefined through discourses and social practices involving relations of power and resistance (Law, 1996, p 44).

Ethnicity and health

The use of ethnicity in health research has been characterised by different approaches according to research aims and the paradigm used.

Approaches that focus on ethnic identity and the meanings surrounding this may operationalise ethnicity in terms of cultural and group affiliations (Nazroo, 1998, p 710). Research into culturally sensitive professional practice, for example, which includes communication, sometimes uses concepts of ethnicity in this way. However, the studies do not always acknowledge the thorny conceptual issues of equating cultural knowledge and sensitivity with untheorised ethnic categories. Some of the research is vulnerable to criticisms of 'racialisation' (Ahmad, 1993, p 19). Racialisation involves the assumption that populations can only meaningfully be divided into 'ethnic' or 'racial' groups, taking these as primary categories for explanatory purposes to the exclusion of other factors. This danger is highlighted for the use of ethnicity in research into communication and culture in health care.

On the other hand, much research has not explicitly theorised ethnicity, but the operational categories have still been criticised for over-generalisation and simplification, and for relying on externally imposed categories without taking adequate account of user categories (Nazroo, 1998, p 713). This applies not only to epidemiological research but also much of the research into communication. The interpretation of data is flawed if based on the assumption that such categories are homogeneous, rather than socially constructed in ways that may obscure differences of history, language, geography, and socio-economic position (Nazroo, 1998, p 713). The use of ethnicity as an independent variable in research is criticised if it leads to claims made on the basis of descriptive correlations that 'ethnic differences' from assumed white 'norms' cause inequalities of outcome in health where there may be multiple causes (Law, 1996, pp 156-7).

Recently, attempts have been made to plot an escape from the research and development traps outlined above. Suggestions include assigning individuals to ethnic categories on the basis of sufficient data, consistency, and dealing with complex realities like 'dual heritage' or 'mixed parentage' (Nazroo, 1998, p 713). One option is to provide respondents with better opportunities and more relevant choices to provide descriptions of their own ethnicity. Also, if ethnicity is treated as an explanatory variable it becomes important to ask not only what it is used to measure, but how its interaction with other potential influences is treated.

Ethnicity and communication

Communication research in particular has been subject to the criticism that definitions of ethnicity tend not to be based on theories, and that social constructs are treated as self-evident social realities, or as unproblematic geopolitical classifications (Leets et al, 1996, p 115). A sizeable proportion of studies fail to report how they measure ethnicity at all (Leets et al, 1996, p 130).

Researching the link between communication and ethnicity requires some consideration of social identity since communication involves individuals interacting within a context shaped by and shaping mutual attributions of social identity. When miscommunication occurs, this can have problematic consequences for health care outcomes. Miscommunication is explained, in the socio-psychological communication literature, in terms of the application of differing mental frameworks for interpreting the relevance of conversational utterances to goals and beliefs (McTear and King, 1991, p 199). Such breakdown may partly derive from tensions, misunderstandings and misattributions over social identity. This, of course, in some cases interacts with further problems connected with language fluency. The place of ethnic identity, in users' and practitioners' views of social identity, needs to be given careful consideration in communication research that is concerned with users who are not fluent in English. Communication research may then seek to explore how "different conceptualisations of ethnicity are linked to different communication practices" (Leets et al, 1996, p 137) by participants in an encounter. For example, communication may be influenced by the extent to which practitioners view aspects of patients' health beliefs and behaviour through the prism of consciously or unconsciously held ideas of ethnicity. This requires, at least, a methodology which accommodates dynamic and fluid concepts of ethnicity, and which seeks out the assessments attached to social categories by different participants in different situations.

In this light, research into ethnicity, communication and health needs to be evaluated partly for the quality with which its operational use of ethnicity is clarified at a conceptual level. In this text, specific studies define ethnicity in a number of different ways, and are evaluated in part for this.

Racism

The concept of racism is highly relevant to any understanding of barriers to access to health care for minority ethnic communities. The 2000 Race Relations (Amendment) Act strengthens the statutory duty for public authorities to examine discriminatory practices and promote racial equality. Yet the explanatory value and the range of meanings associated with the concept are contested, with attempts to distinguish between different levels and workings of racism in different situations and with different ethnic communities.

In general, current debates concern the use of restricted or expanded definitions of racism. Restricted definitions seek to exclude a range of implicit or indirect attributions which might lead to weakened opportunities to obtain evidence, and to the confounding of racism with other possible factors influencing offensive behaviour, for example gender or class bias. This restricted definition rests on the two ideas of 'marking race' and of 'negative attribution' (Miles, 1989; Law, 1996), which excludes a great range of potentially racially motivated behaviour of an indirect kind, tied to social or institutional structures and practices. One justification for the restricted definition is that it removes the difficulty of establishing 'unintended' racism as, nevertheless, racist.

Expanded definitions seek to include indirect racism, and a crucial example of this is the concept of institutional racism.

Problems accompany the attempt to exclude the unintended or indirect forms. Intentions are hard to demonstrate, especially with the ambiguity surrounding utterances concerning ethnic differences. More generally, a shift of emphasis away from intentions to effects has been motivated in part by the concern to develop legislative and policy frameworks which locate ultimate responsibility for practice within collective social organisation rather than, solely, individual behaviour.

An expanded notion of racism attempts to operationalise the concepts of institutional and indirect racism. Such an expanded version connects particular practices to underlying mechanisms within social organisations that give rise to or perpetuate such practices.

The UK Commission for Racial Equality (CRE) states that "institutional racism has been defined as those established laws, customs and practices which systematically reflect and produce racial inequalities in society". By this CRE definition, "organisational structures, policies, processes and practices which result in ethnic minorities being treated unfairly and less equally, often without intention or knowledge" are institutionally racist (MacPherson Report, 1999, 6.30).

The MacPherson Report applies the following concept of institutional racism:

> The collective failure of an organisation to provide an appropriate and professional service to people because of their colour, culture, or ethnic origin. It can be seen or detected in processes, attitudes and behaviour which amount to discrimination through unwitting prejudice, ignorance, thoughtlessness and racist stereotyping which disadvantage minority ethnic people. (MacPherson Report, 1999, 6.34)

In this context, the 2000 Race Relations (Amendment) Act apparently provides a powerful legislative driver for change in health service institutions. For example, institutions might be held accountable for inertia in provision of communication resources to overcome the inequitable effects of provision. However, while such an approach clearly seeks to achieve institutional change, difficulties have been identified. The main problem with using expanded definitions is to establish evidence of a causal link between organisational structures, policies and processes, and specific instances of practice. There are a number of related difficulties – the possibilities of multiple causes of a particular problem, the difficulties of obtaining evidence, and the implications of resistance and denial. It is also difficult to establish the link between an effect in terms of measures of equity based on social need and its cause in practice.

When reviewing the evidence from any health research that considers racism, several questions may be important. First, is the concept used operationally, or peripherally, in the context of research, which may operationalise other terms such as, for example, 'cultural sensitivity'? Second, if racism is not operationalised is this a significant omission? Third, does the research define racism within a restricted or expanded framework? Fourth, if there is operationalisation of racism, is it adequate to the conceptual framework used and the problems raised?

Racism and health

In health research specifically, the overall framework within which the research is conducted, and the language and terminology used, are significant to the validity of the study. As we have seen, it has been argued that the concentration of health research in certain areas at the expense of others sometimes constitutes an example of 'racialisation' (Ahmad, 1993, p 17). The concept of racialisation draws on an expanded definition of racism, focusing on effects rather than intentions of discourse, without which the issues and methods of health research on minority ethnic communities, and the ways in which the boundaries of such research are drawn and redrawn, could not be questioned.

Concerning the focus and content of the research, a restricted definition of racism remains relevant to the analysis of direct and specific communication behaviours, for example face-to-face encounters, while an expanded definition, which may be relevant to specific communication behaviours, is also relevant to issues of service provision and effects. Direct racism is perhaps implicated in empirical studies which show that GPs consider, despite conflicting evidence, that Asians consult more frequently with trivial complaints, demand longer consultations and are less compliant (Smaje, 1995, pp 109–11). In this case, the use of cultural stereotypes provides simplistic explanations to complex issues involving communication difficulties. But assessing the implications of this for policy depends on the use of expanded definitions, looking at effects of attitudes and their interaction with collective policy and provision, for example in the use of interpreting services.

The conceptual challenge for research and development is to clarify whether, and how, recognised barriers to communication can be identified as involving racist practice. A number of recurring themes emerge from a literature search into issues of communication and access to health care for users who lack fluency in English. Among these are:

- inadequate consultation to identify the needs of disadvantaged communities;
- inequitable referrals across a complex system;
- inadequate provision of properly trained interpreters, linkworkers and advocates;
- shortcomings in the use of information such as translated and audio-visual materials for health promotion;
- problems of miscommunication in consultations with or without interpreters;
- stereotypical cultural attitudes and beliefs influencing communication.

Clearly, it is easier to obtain empirical evidence of any of these issues and problems at an individual level, and to implement interventions at the same level designed to enhance communication, than it is to design research that would produce robust evidence showing that the problems at an individual level are attributable to institutional factors and therefore demand collective attention.

There are also important overlaps between practices which may be deemed racist and other gatekeeping communicative practices in health care which facilitate or sustain differential access to resources. For example, differential practice was said to impact on the way doctors communicate with parents of children with Down's syndrome compared with the way they communicate with other parents, in a study of practice at a paediatric cardiology clinic (Silverman, 1987, pp 137–8). The practice may involve selective framing and communication of information, or non-communication of information, in individual consultations or collective health promotion. The point is significant because the focus of research into minority ethnic health care users who lack fluency in English could, if handled in a purely contrastive way, against a mythical white norm, contribute to the marginalisation and indeed racialisation of that research. The significant overlaps with other differential communicative practices can be clarified by comparative as well as contrastive analysis.

In sum, the concept of racism is complex, and the demonstration of indirect racism is problematic. Yet the importance of conceptual clarity in defining and identifying different forms of racism is evident, for understanding inequities in health care policy and practice involving communication. At the same time, research that takes account of racist communication policy and practice should be conducted in the context of a broader concern with identifying the mechanisms that support all differential and exclusionary practices.

Culture

Concepts of cultural difference and health beliefs

The most significant models of culture that have been used in health research are summarised below. These models conceptualise 'difference' in diverse ways, with diverse results. Perhaps the most widespread approach applies a concept of 'cultural difference' to either the examination of causes of ill health in populations or the investigation of the meanings different ethnic communities attribute to health and well-being. This overall approach has, however, sometimes been adopted in a problematic manner. It has then been criticised for its influence on methodologies, in comparing ways of life of minority ethnic communities (viewed as a possible cause of problems) with 'white' norms, and for its over-simplistic application (Culley, 1996, p 568; Lambert and Sivak, 1996, pp 124-8).

The use of cultural difference does not necessarily imply acknowledgement of the many complexities of cultural diversity. In one apparently conservative view, culture is defined as a shared system of meanings, values and ways of life that emerge from group experience and are transmitted from one generation to another" (Chu, 1998, p 126). Such a view tends to present culture as static – a baton passed on from generation to generation. The resulting belief, shown, for example, in some transcultural nursing literature, is that research can catalogue enduring 'differences' in terms of universal human values and behaviours and culture–restricted ones (Leininger, 1984). In pioneering a transcultural nursing movement, Leininger (p 42) cites 173 "care constructs" for more than 50 cultures. This approach, though clearly useful on some levels, has been criticised for ignoring structural aspects of culture (Papadopoulos and Alleyne, 1998, p 3). It may underestimate how elements of specific cultures can achieve wider cultural currency. Such elements may also undergo changes under changing structural, socio-economic, and historic influences. The approach may also, by tending to tie culture to ethnicity, ignore the impact of other variables like gender, age and socio-economic status on health beliefs.

At worst, empirical studies may draw on static notions of cultural difference in values and practices without involving users in the research at any stage, and then seek to illuminate patterns of behaviour by accounting for them in stereotypical terms of negative cultural attributes. For example, a US study of cross-cultural differences in the care of patients with cancer illustrates differences of sex roles with an example of a man with cancer whose habitual infidelity is attributed to "the macho role typical of certain cultures" (Trill and Holland, 1993, p 22).

Evidence deriving from over-simplistic research may then reinforce negative aspects of practice rather than underpinning best practice. Stereotypes of difference may impede professional practice as well as research, by being superimposed simplistically as an explanatory framework onto patterns of interaction that they then may reinforce. Specific interactional patterns of talk used by health professionals and service users can differ in a number of ways whether or not both parties are speaking English. For example, the use of silences, overlaps, and intonation patterns may differ, as may patterns of talk expressing politeness, in ways that reflect factors such as power as well as cultural and language difference. The 'intercultural' situation may then be compounded by differing interpretations of the communication problems that arise, which generate further communication problems. For instance, in a study of views of health professionals in Melbourne, Australia (Pauwels, 1990), cultural differences in patterns for structuring oral interactions are complex, and perhaps to some extent fostered by stereotype-like perceptions by health professionals that:

"... their questions are very direct, almost abrupt."

"... they are not familiar with our meeting routines...."

"... you should have a few pleasantries to start your consultation with the patient, ...they [the patients] don't seem able to do that." (Pauwels, 1990, p 103)

The comments illustrate how differences in frameworks of knowledge for speech events are all too easily accounted for by stereotypes with a moral dimension ("you should have"), which may reinforce or partly account for the behavioural patterns in question. The extent to which such stereotyping is encouraged within specific organisational cultures has not been adequately researched.

Allowing for diversity

There are, however, better alternative models for research. To draw together recurrent strands emerging from a review of recent empirical work, several conceptual issues underlie operational definitions of culture (as debated elsewhere, for example in Ahmad, 1996, pp 190–219; Kelleher, 1996, pp 69–90). These conceptual issues all concern the extent to which the research frames 'difference' in terms which allow for complexity-in-diversity. One issue is how dynamic or static the concept is, taking into account the integration of new and older cultural patterns under specific social and economic influences (Lambert and Sivak, 1996, pp 124–59). Another concern is how far the model of culture used accounts for the difference between statements of belief or attitude, and behaviour in specific contexts (Ahmad, 1996, p 203). A third issue is how broad or narrow the scope of cultural practice is, for example whether simply related to ethnicity and notions of ethno-cultural difference, or also encompassing professional and institutional cultures, as in the health service (Guarnaccia and Rodriguez, 1996, pp 419–37). A further problem is how far the model accommodates the tension between self-definitions and external definitions (Kelleher, 1996, p 78). The main focus in this section will be on the issue of dynamism as a major factor in cultural diversity.

The extent to which definitions of culture incorporate dynamism has far-reaching effects for research. At the same time, a more dynamic approach to cultural diversity must take account of a number of issues that have been highlighted in the literature (for example in Guarnaccia and Rodriguez, 1996, pp 419–37; Lambert and Sivak, 1996, p 148; L. Robinson, 1998, pp 4–64), some of which are briefly summarised here. Patterns of migration impact on cultural developments in communities.

Generational differences influence beliefs and behaviours. Structural factors impact on cultural changes, for example with health service reforms affecting cultures within health service organisations. There are also internal differentiations of gender, and socio-economic background within cultures associated with specific ethnic communities. Biculturalism involves the embracing of cultural values from different traditions, and acculturation involves the gradual shift of marginalised cultures towards a mainstream culture. There is also a dynamic tension between the influence of self-determination and the influence of external categorisation on cultural identities. Lastly, with situational variation, cultural practices vary according to context, for example in different institutional settings. Several of these issues may, of course, interact.

The concept of acculturation may be treated with mistrust if its research use is exclusively in terms of the shift of beliefs and behaviours of minority ethnic health users towards the mainstream. However, a more complex research strategy might investigate the extent to which professionals as well as patients are influenced by acculturation, and the strategies professionals may use to manage conflicts which may arise. In Guarnaccia and Rodriguez's (1996) analysis:

> ... thus dominant cultural norms and values are built into the frameworks for the training of professionals, for assessment of clients, and for developing treatment approaches. (Guarnaccia and Rodriguez, 1996, p 432)

Also, practitioners may be powerfully influenced by workplace cultures, as

> ... professionals generally work within institutional frameworks that have their own cultures. (Guarnaccia and Rodriguez, 1996, p 432)

In addition, there is the issue of breadth and scope of definition. As Guarnaccia and Rodriguez indicate, definitions of culture may limit the scope to the management of everyday behavioural or life-world problems:

> ... culture provides a variety of resources for dealing with major life changes and challenges, including serious illness and hospitalisation. (Guarnaccia and Rodriguez, 1996, p 437)

On the other hand, they may broaden the scope to include legislative frameworks, institutionalised custom, literature, etc (Kelleher, 1996, p 71). The broader scope provides a better framework for analysing service policy and its implementation.

Research into communication and health also needs to find ways of interpreting the impact of gender-related and age-related cultural identities as well as ethnic-related and professional or institutional cultural identities. Discourses around age, gender and ethnicity provide 'organising' conceptual frameworks (Kelleher, 1996, p 76), which may influence choices for cultural self-definition and other-definition.

This section has indicated that the value of any research studies must depend in part on how culture is operationally defined in illuminating its potential influences on practice. This definition needs to take account of various aspects of dynamism, of the breadth and diversity of culture, and the distinction between external and self-definition.

Communication and culture

The importance of effective interpersonal relations and of evidence-based practice is widely emphasised in the contemporary health service (Barker, 2000, p 329). However, the quality of research evidence on interpersonal communication across boundaries of language, culture and ethnicity depends in part on matters of conceptual underpinning. This section discusses research approaches that specifically investigate communication and culture, and then refers to models of transcultural communication competence which have been proposed for professional practice, but not empirically evaluated. Much of the research into communication, culture and health has been carried out within sociological frameworks of enquiry (Martin and Nakayama, 1999, pp 2-3). As far as research into face-to-face communication is concerned, two approaches have predominated.

In one positivist approach, group membership and related cultural patterns are used to predict communicative behaviour (Martin and Nakayama, 1999, p 4). Here the focus is on cultural difference as an explanatory variable. This approach focuses on orderly and stable characteristics of culture, and usually imposes externally predefined categories of meaning on events (Martin and Nakayama, 1999, p 4). It does not easily take account of dynamic cross-currents of individual cultural affiliations, nor does it lend itself to close analysis of how communication is shaped across turns of talk.

The second approach, an interpretative paradigm has the goal of interpreting rather than predicting behaviour, and culture is viewed as socially constructed and emergent. The meanings attributed to events by participants are viewed as actively contributing to knowledge. Research is often conducted, at least in part, from an insider or 'emic' perspective, while the relationship between culture and communication may be mutually reinforcing (Martin and Nakayama, 1999, p 6).

Miscommunication and culture

Within the interpretative paradigm, a fascinating body of research has focused on miscommunication and culture. The interactional socio-linguistic perspective assumes that different strategies for talk and different communication styles, although influenced by different cultural and ethnic backgrounds, are at the core of miscommunication (Sarangi, 1994, p 411). This approach (Gumperz, 1982; Scollon and Scollon, 1995; Roberts, 1998), encourages close empirical analysis of sequences of talk, though ultimately, again, attributing miscommunication to cultural difference. Linguistic features, for example special intonation features, pitch choices, or word or idiom choices, such as 'yes' or 'mm' or *silence* as a response, which trigger off background knowledge used by listeners for making inferences about meanings, can be interpreted differently by speakers and listeners across cultural boundaries, and this, it is assumed, leads to conversational troubles. Differences might consist, for example, in assigning an information meaning to an expression like 'right' where an interpersonal meaning is more important, or vice-versa. A criticism of this approach is that misunderstanding of such features may as easily derive from a person's unfamiliarity with institutional norms, or from gender differences, as from ethnicity-related cultural differences (Sarangi, 1994, p 412). It also leaves unexamined the extent to which differences of cultural beliefs and attitudes may contribute to miscommunication regardless of linguistic features. Practitioners and patients, for example, may attribute communication problems to essential cultural and attitudinal differences and so exacerbate the problems, regardless of their actual causes. For non-fluent speakers, such factors may also interact with basic comprehension and production difficulties of grammar and vocabulary, and pressures on language processing such as time limits. It seems clear, in fact, that health research is needed that takes due account of the complexities of communication on several levels.

Communication and health

As regards sociologically influenced research in the field of health and communication, it has been argued that several models have been used (Hyden and Mishler, 1999, pp 174-92). These models are:

- a 'speaking-to-patients' model which focuses on clinical communication techniques;
- a 'speaking-with-patients' model which focuses on two-way or multi-party interaction;
- a 'speaking-about-patients' model which focuses on professional discourses about illness;
- a 'speaking-by-patients' model which focuses on patients' illness and recovery narratives.

The speaking-to-patients model

The speaking-to-patients model focuses on identifying categories of talk which health professionals may use instrumentally to enhance communication across the professional–client divide (Roter and Hall, 1989). This model isolates predefined categories of talk abstracted from the ebb and flow of turn-by-turn interaction. Applied to communication across boundaries of language and ethnicity, it tends to focus on enumerating techniques for carrying out clinical tasks and ensuring compliance.

The speaking-with-patients model

The speaking-with-patients model focuses on the sequences of exchanges between clinical professionals and patients, and identifies the communicative functions of different recurrent patterns of institutional talk. This approach is of particular interest, since the focus is on patients and professionals interacting at the sharp end of communication where impressions that endure can be managed and mismanaged. Interactional patterns of turn-taking shaping of talk in relation to prior utterances, linguistic signalling of expectations for talk, and conventions of topic management are interpreted in the light of asymmetries of power and cultural knowledge (Hyden and Mishler, 1999, p 176-82). It becomes possible to focus comparatively on different speech styles used recurrently in different institutional contexts, and on the different contexts in which discrepancies in communication occur (Heritage and Sefi, 1992). Institutional cultural norms are revealed as they recurrently influence patterns of communication (Silverman, 1987). The approach reveals different strategies of communication which accomplish medical agendas in specific institutional contexts, for example the strategic use of a series of question-and-answer sequences across a series of 'turns' where practitioner and patient alternate in speaking (Maynard, 1992).

A speaking-with-patients approach also has the potential to provide much-needed evidence concerning communication between practitioners, patients who are not fluent in English, and family members or professional interpreters. In multi-party transcultural communication, problems may arise through aspects of inaccurate translation and through misunderstandings about participant roles. Studies have shown, for example, that translation may alter information or relationship messages by omission of detail, substitution of one concept for another, conceptual simplification or condensation of a complicated response, interchanging closed and open questioning (Farooq et al, 1997, p 211), and addition of information (Hornberger et al, 1996, p 849). The speaking-with-patients may be used alone, or with other approaches, as described below, to explore the dynamics of such multi-party interactions.

The speaking-about-patients model

Research into discourses 'about' patients may focus on different cultural levels, for example policy documents, journal science, and professional, workplace cultures, and investigate these as possible influences on interactions with patients (Lupton, 1994; Atkinson, 1995). Research may even focus at a macro level on the way in which research models of 'health communication' are linked to or influenced by health policy agendas.

The speaking-by-patients model

Research using the speaking-by-patients model focuses on the patients' own narratives of their lives in relation to illness and health, and examines the social (for example familial) contexts which influence their talk (Good and Good, 1994; Hyden and Mishler, 1999, pp 179-84). Such an approach can illuminate how cultural and individual meaning is sustained under the threat of illness.

Linkages between research models

An important consideration is possible linkages between speaking-with-patients, speaking-about-patients and speaking-by-patients approaches. So research into consultation processes 'with patients' should perhaps be strengthened by a discourse analysis locating the interactional patterns of words, values and concepts within a broader framework of social processes and institutional cultures, values and practices (Lupton, 1994, p 61).

Research into the way practitioners and family member/carers or professional interpreters speak with and about patients who are not fluent in English might productively be combined with exploration of the words spoken by patients themselves. Using such an approach, and perhaps combining interviews with direct observational methods, researchers can explore some of the complexities of communication between practitioners, patients and their carers, and, perhaps, bilingual liaison workers such as advocates and linkworkers, or interpreters. Much remains to be understood about the widespread use of family members as interpreters in primary care, for example. Here, issues of language production, understanding and translation, interpersonal rapport, and perceptions of roles, beliefs, attitudes and values concerning health, all converge. Dilemmas of confidentiality, and of provision of support for patients in confronting power differences, come to the fore. In such contexts, the management of divided attention, where, for example, practitioners must attend to both patient and interpreter, can affect information and relationship quality. These areas are under-researched, especially regarding views of different parties in relation to the information content and relationship aspects. A combined speaking-with-patients, speaking-by-patients and speaking-about-patients approach to research might involve a combination of observational and interview methods to inform evidence-based practice in this area.

In sum, there may be advantages in research taking a combined approach in order to illuminate some of the intricate processes of transcultural communication, without neglecting the influences of social and cultural contexts. The advantages of not restricting research to a speaking-to-patients orientation include that of preventing a narrow focus on cultural difference which can emphasise adaptive techniques and problem cultures in a way that reinforces misleading stereotypes.

Transcultural communication competence

It might be expected that the issues involved in conceptualising cultural diversity and communication would be reflected not only in research approaches but in frameworks used for assessing practitioner competence. However, there is no existing, empirically evaluated blueprint for effective transcultural communication. For example, an influential model views cultural awareness, cultural knowledge and cultural sensitivity as attributes of transcultural competence (Papadopoulos et al, 1998), but makes no explicit reference to communication as a central concept.

A theoretical 'competence' framework, integrating knowledge and skills, is presented by Gerrish et al (1996, pp 26–31), drawing heavily on Kim (1992), in the context of an evaluation of educational programmes. Cultural communicative competence is viewed as the ability to understand cultural patterns, rules for interaction and behavioural patterns of specific cultures (Gerrish et al, 1996, p 26). This can be viewed as a knowledge component. Intercultural communicative competence is viewed as a set of communicative skills which enable individuals to suspend or modify their own cultural expectations and to be able to accommodate to new cultural demands (Gerrish et al, 1996, pp 27-9). The skills involve elements of cognitive flexibility, affective empathy and behavioural adaptability, and can be integrated in performance. Both cultural knowledge and intercultural skills are important, as 'transcultural communicative competence' involves the ability to use and modify knowledge through generic communicative skills. This knowledge and skills training model envisages such 'competence' as developing through stages from 'unconscious incompetence', through consciousness of limitations, to a degree of unconscious automaticity (Gerrish et al, 1996, p 31). However, the place of reflection in developing competence, and in preventing practitioners' behaviour becoming so 'automatic' and routine-governed that this may result in blunted sensitivity and, perhaps, thereby underpin depersonalising or stereotyping practices, is not clearly modelled. Also, the emphasis on skills is not fleshed out with a focus on practice conditions, or language issues.

A comparable transcultural communication competence model is that of Gudykunst and Kim (1992a). This model includes three interrelated dimensions: skills, motivation, and knowledge. It also includes socio-cognitive elements, which are viewed as facilitative of gains in the three dimensions. One element of the model involves becoming cognitively 'mindful' in action, or, perhaps, reflective, in order to adapt ones thinking and feelings and be open to new perspectives. Another element involves developing behavioural flexibility, and a tolerance for ambiguity and uncertainty, in order to reduce anxiety in communication. Drawing on this model, an implication of highlighting 'mindfulness' is that practitioner self-awareness might be viewed as an important facet of transcultural communication competence, taking account, for example, of the possible influence on practice of subconsciously held attitudes towards particular patient groups.

Such theoretical models would benefit from development through empirical evaluation. A concern, in reviewing empirical communication research involving service users who are not fluent in English, is how rarely the studies question what transculturally competent communication might involve, for individuals or organisations, and how it might be measured in terms of practice processes and outcomes.

To summarise this section, published transcultural communication competence models give consideration to skills, knowledge, attitudes and, underpinning these three, reflective ability or 'mindfulness'. Competence also implies a capacity to assess service environments and to act on organisational and practical constraints as they affect communication.

As this study turns to describe and evaluate the empirical research on barriers to communication between minority ethnic service users and providers, and then the interventions which have aimed to enhance communication, a significant aspect of the evaluation concerns how the research uses key concepts discussed in this chapter *operationally*. There are a number of key issues to consider. These include:

- the extent to which conceptual rigour is sustained through the empirical work;
- the ways in which social context and structure are handled;
- the ways in which the chosen methodologies encourage evidence of relevant complexities of communication processes and outcomes to emerge.

Notes

[1] The term 'minority ethnic' is preferred to 'ethnic minority' since the use of the latter term would imply a contrast reinforcing the impression that some populations (for example, a 'white' majority in the UK) are not defined on the basis of ethnicity.

[2] Fluency refers to the ability of a person to communicate easily, rapidly and continuously in a particular language (Crystal, 1987, p 278). Such fluency involves combining many skills at once (K. Johnson, 1996, p 42), when listening, understanding or speaking. Included among those skills are adhering to grammatical and vocabulary norms, negotiating semantic meanings (understandings), relating to socially expected norms concerning role relationships, and relating to what another person is saying (coherence). Lack of fluency is a matter of degree, and speakers may in practice display different degrees of fluency in different contexts and under different pressures.

Part one:
Communication barriers

Introduction

In recent years, with growing realisation of the extent of cultural and language variation among minority ethnic users of the health service, it has also been acknowledged that viewpoints of minority ethnic patients have not been well understood, and that in some situations their needs are not met adequately (Vydelingum, 2000, p 100; Gerrish, 2001). Within this context, the specific communication needs of patients who are not fluent in English need to be identified and addressed. As was noted in the Introduction, government White Papers and current NHS educational policy support action on addressing the needs of minority ethnic users (*Saving lives: Our healthier nation*, 1999; *Clinical governance*, 1999; *Making a difference*, 1999). However, the documents make few explicit references to communication issues, so that the full extent of communication barriers to effective practice remains to be acknowledged at policy level.

Despite the policy initiatives, there is abundant evidence that the health service and health practitioners do not always meet the communication needs of minority ethnic patients effectively. Clearly, communication problems persist between practitioners and minority ethnic patients at an individual face-to-face level. For example, Vydelingum (2000) claims that "studies on utilisation of hospital services by South Asian patients have consistently demonstrated levels of dissatisfaction with communication and language difficulties" (p 101). Such issues have widespread application and can threaten disclosure, informed consent, (McNamara at al, 1997, pp 361-3) and health outcomes.

There is also evidence to suggest that structural factors exist and contribute to poor communication with minority ethnic patients. As a result of failures of organisation, resource management and planning, access to health services and utilisation are often problematic (Gerrish, 2000). The barriers which have been identified include, for example, the lack of bilingual services at the point of need (Lam and Green, 1994; Farshi et al, 1999), inadequate monitoring of ethnicity (Lawrenson et al, 1998) and poor use of referral systems (Arora et al, 1995). Finally, inadequate use of information resources can be a barrier to user participation.

The next two chapters aim to provide a summary account of some of the most significant process and structural barriers in these areas, so as to inform the subsequent evaluation of interventions. The first chapter explores communication process barriers, focusing on the adaptation of prevailing practice models to transcultural communication contexts, stereotyping, and language and miscommunication.

ONE

Process barriers

Adaptation of prevailing models to transcultural communication contexts

Different perceptions of care influence communication processes whether or not any cultural differences are accurately recognised. Nevertheless, greater awareness of caring models can lead to more effective communication strategies. Nursing educational courses in the UK, for example, encourage health practitioners to engage in some form of activity that promotes holistic care (Sourial, 1997) and patient empowerment (Rodwell, 1996). Looking at nurses' conceptualisation of individualised care within a multi-ethnic society, Gerrish (2000) identifies important tenets such as promoting independence, partnership and negotiation of care, and equity. There also appears to be a deepening consensus of opinion on the importance of transcultural models (Gerrish et al, 1996; Papadopoulos et al, 1998). These models have the potential to enhance health care practice.

However, the application of such models by practitioners may involve engagement with obstacles and struggle. This is partly in response to communication difficulties where patients feel unable to interact with practitioners due to language barriers (Gerrish, 2001). There may be tensions between the ideologies of individualised care as practised by health professionals and the health beliefs of minority ethnic communities who may view health problems as to some degree a collective rather than an individual responsibility (Gerrish, 2000). Indeed, research evidence indicates significant barriers in the application of prevailing models.

In general, professionals' views of particular problems are influenced by their beliefs about practice. In the nursing profession, communication difficulties in caring for minority ethnic patients who lack fluency in English may be viewed as obstacles to the provision of holistic care and the development of a therapeutic relationship. For example, one qualitative interview study of the views of 18 nurses about caring for minority ethnic patients in the UK found that all respondents viewed communication as their biggest challenge (Murphy and Macleod Clark, 1993, p 444).

Interestingly, the majority of nurses portrayed difficulties in forming affective relationships with clients, for example:

> "I don't feel as if I got to know her or to understand how she was feeling. I didn't feel I had a relationship, it was purely on a clinical basis." (cited in Murphy and Macleod Clark, 1993, p 445)

From the nurses' perspectives, in the Murphy and Macleod Clark study, the main cause of relationship difficulties appeared to be communication problems, partly because of lack of cultural knowledge and more specifically because of language problems.

In similar vein, a recent ethnographic study conducted by Gerrish (2001) focused on 22 district nurses attempting to care holistically for 221 South Asian patients. The findings demonstrated that the nurses' practice showed "several ways in which patients who spoke little English were disadvantaged" (Gerrish, 2001, p 571). For example, "a daily dressing to a surgical wound on an elderly Indian woman who spoke only Hindi was undertaken competently by the nurses but they could provide little additional care" (Gerrish 2001, p 571). The interpersonal fluidity between the nurses and the patient seemed to be restricted, as no one was available to interpret at the point of care provision.

When there are interpersonal difficulties in areas such as these, it is likely that holistic care will be compromised. Situations will be distorted and perceived with less realism and patient choice and negotiation of care will be severely impaired. Yet the patients in this study, who spoke little English, were rarely asked whether they wanted an interpreter, apparently at least in part due to the expressed concern by the nurses that this could detract from their relationship with the patient.

The majority of respondents in the Murphy and Macleod Clark study stated frequent feelings of frustration in dealing with minority ethnic patients. The inability to form a relationship and to provide holistic rather than physical care generated stress:

> "It's quite stressful sometimes. You know when you are looking after someone, you want to look after them wholly and you can't."
> (cited in Murphy and Macleod Clark, 1993, pp 447-8)

Respondents who attributed the frustration of their professional aspirations through communication and cultural barriers reported reacting by a withdrawal into a more limited form of physical task-orientated care rather than holistic care (Murphy and Macleod Clark, 1993, p 449). Such a role restriction could be frustrating and have further attitudinal consequences both for nurses and patients. To overcome this, a professional model of culturally competent caring may need to encompass the potential roles of bilingual professionals, and relatives, in enhancing a satisfactory level of communication.

A further example of barriers to the provision of individual care is brought into focus by Vydelingum (2000). In a qualitative study using a purposive sample of 10 patients in acute care and six carers, altogether five Hindus, five Sikhs and six Muslims, patient isolation was highlighted. The findings indicated that patients often felt they were 'passing through' and 'alone in a crowd', trying to 'fit in'. The 'alone in a crowd' theme focuses on communication difficulties and illuminates extreme isolation reported by patients due to the language barrier. For instance:

> "I have to wait for my daughter to come so she could tell the nurse or doctor. There were no interpreters; I did not think you could ask for interpreters, I feel terrible that I could not speak to the nurses, so lonely." (Vydelingum, 2000, p 103)

The communication difficulties seemed exacerbated by the nurse's lack of positive action in providing resources to facilitate effective communication. Nurses were also perceived as busy and not responding appropriately to patient needs; for example, information about diagnosis, medication and discharge were often insufficient (Vydelingum, 2000, p 104).

A further concern in the application of prevailing models is that practitioners and patients may have different perceptions of the caring paradigm. In the practical application of caring models, practitioners' expectation of patient involvement seems to be high, in terms of supplying information about health problems, in goal-setting and the implementation of treatment programmes. On the other hand, if language constraints exist or cultural beliefs differ, the patient may not respond in a way that matches practitioner demands. Yet there is evidence of ambivalent attitudes from some practitioners to various coping strategies which may enhance patient involvement and empowerment, such as use of family members, and bilingual interpreters or linkworkers (Murphy and MacLeod Clark, 1993, p 446-9). An underlying issue is that practitioners may need to re-evaluate some of their tenets concerning patient autonomy in the light of a better and non-stereotypical understanding of the views of minority ethnic patients concerning identity, health, and treatment plans (Phipps, 1995). Examples would include patient views on maternal recuperation after childbirth, and on familial involvement in issues of disclosure and informed consent.

Communication problems may arise when over-individualistic models of autonomy, or conversely, over-simplistic, stereotypical models of cultural and familial dependence, are applied in health care. The stereotypical view that families 'cope' is sometimes used by practitioners to account for low knowledge and use of health services by South Asians, and this can reinforce an element of inertia in terms of outreach activities, with evidence, for example, of low referral rates of South Asian patients to community health services by some doctors (Ritch et al 1996, p 220).

The studies outlined in this section represent a state of affairs where the diverse needs of individual patients are, at times, poorly met. Although the transcultural paradigm is concerned with delivering high standards of care, barriers of particular intractability persist, involving the residue of depersonalising and disempowering traditions and practices. It must be recognised that, to embrace diversity, practitioners need the skills, awareness and commitment to consult with patients about their communication wants, and to seek support as and when appropriate.

Stereotyping

A significant barrier to dialogue between professionals and patients is that of stereotyping. The 'intercultural' situation may be compounded by differing interpretations of communication difficulties, which generate yet more problems. For example, in a study of views of health professionals in Melbourne (Pauwels, 1990), cultural differences in patterns for structuring oral interactions are complex and perhaps to some extent fostered by stereotype-like perceptions of patients by health professionals, such as:

"... their questions are very direct, almost abrupt."

"... you should have a few pleasantries to start your consultation with the patient ... they don't seem able to do that." (Pauwels, 1990, p 103)

The comments illustrate how differences in frameworks of knowledge for speech events are all too easily accounted for by stereotypes with a moral dimension ("you should have"), which may reinforce or partly account for the behavioural patterns in question.

Ideas similar to those put forward by Pauwels are to be found in the work of Bowler (1993) on the attitudes of 25 British midwives to South Asian women. Stereotypes of 'Asian' women who are not interested in or compliant with services, and consequently abuse them, were mobilised to account for communication difficulties. Women's expressions were sometimes interpreted as signs of rudeness. Some women did not say 'please' or 'thank you' and seemed to be 'giving orders' (Bowler, 1993, p 11). Midwives in this study reported that Asian women were not interested in contraception advice and abused the service by having large families.

This stereotypical account justified instances of differential practice, such as a midwife's reluctance to explore possibilities of contraception as she was seen to do with other women (Bowler, 1993, p12). Typifying South Asian patients for failure to fulfil normative maternal role expectations again suggests a process of depersonalisation.

The use of cultural stereotypes, strengthened by communicatively problematic experiences with a few individuals, might then be applied by some professionals to a whole, externally imposed ethnic category like 'Asians', without adequately recognising individual and socio-cultural differences:

> "… what we need is an A4 bit of paper with it all on so we can look things up when we need them." (Bowler, 1993, p 15)

Where such depersonalising, stereotyping processes influence equity of provision, this can be seen as racist in effect. The MacPherson Report, which was discussed in the earlier section on racism, identified that institutional racism needs to be related not to conscious intentions but effects (p 6.28). Prejudices of many kinds may influence health care practice, but the 2000 Race Relations (Amendment) Act now places an obligation on the health service to combat discriminatory practices with renewed vigilance.

This section has considered ways in which stereotyping contributes to miscommunication. The next section focuses on culture and gender.

Culture, gender and communication styles

The relationship between gender and culture is a controversial issue in communication. Most research into communication barriers in this area concerns women, not only regarding family and community communicative norms, where for example the attitude of a husband or of a community leader may be significant in sanctioning a women's choices, but also regarding consultation between an individual female patient and a male or female doctor. The scarcity of gender research into minority ethnic males and communication is quite striking.

In primary health care the gender issue differentiates Asian women's experiences of GPs from their experience of nursing professionals, for example district nurses, midwives and health visitors. Claims have been made that South Asian women express a stronger preference for female doctors than women in general (Bowes and Domokos 1995a, pp 29-30). Women who are not fluent in English may then face interacting communication difficulties. Asian women may feel unable to speak with male doctors about intimate concerns, for example childbirth, because of the barriers posed by medical expertise and patriarchy, and because of cultural and gender-related emotions such as embarrassment (Bowes and Domokos 1995a, p 30). To patriarchy and medical dominance must be added the possibility that class differences and ethnic differences also inhibit talk (Bowes and Domokos 1995a, p 30).

Yet, while some studies find a preference by South Asian women for female doctors (Bowes and Domokos 1995b, pp 22-33; McAvoy and Raza, 1988, pp 11-16 – see Ahmad et al 1991), others found a greater tendency for 'Asian' women to prefer a male of the same ethnicity than a female of different ethnicity (Ahmad et al, 1991, p 331). This inconsistency in findings suggests that caution should be observed before generalising findings about a specific ethnic community to another one, and in not underestimating possible significant determinants of attitudes such as age, education level, and social class.

There are reasons to be wary of over-interpreting research on patterns of preference by ethnicity and gender. For example, Bowes and Domokos (1995b) interviewed 20 South Asian Muslim women aged between 26 and 41 in Glasgow; 15 had been born in Pakistan, three in the UK, one in Kenya, and one in Libya. The sample frame is open to question, as:

> ... the interviewees were contacted using a network of personal relationships. (Bowes and Domokos, 1995b, p 147)

Such an approach has the possible disadvantage of representing viewpoints selectively. Questions must therefore be asked about the generalisability of findings to Indian-born or British-born Hindu women, or to Bangladeshi women in the UK.

Related problems are found in the quantitative Bradford study of 1,633 consultations at a general practice (Ahmad et al, 1991, p 330). While the study suggests that selection of practitioner by language and ethnicity may override gender, the methodology not only leaves unaddressed issues about how women patients select GPs, but also about the sample. The category 'Asian' is not refined for doctor or patients except that the patients were "mainly of Pakistani and Indian origin" (Ahmad et al, 1991). An issue here is that the researchers were hampered by the lack of ethnic information on patient records.

Nevertheless, concerns about gender and choice appear to be widely confirmed. For example, a survey of the communication experiences of 500 members of the Asian community with health services in Blackburn (Shah and Piracha, 1993) found that, with regard to feelings about being examined by a doctor of the opposite sex, 87.5% of Asian males were not embarrassed or uncomfortable, compared with 47.7% of Asian females who were either embarrassed or uncomfortable (pp 20-1). Asked about preferences for service improvement, over 90% of the Asian sample also said that more female health professionals should be available, compared with only 57.5% for a white control group (p 24). Concern about the shortage of available female GPs was widespread among Asian women. Similarly, a survey at the A&E department of Birmingham Heartlands hospital found that, whereas 85% of 41 'white' females did not mind the gender of their doctor, only 52% of 125 minority ethnic female patients did not mind (Karim, 1996, pp 77-8).

Despite the difficulties in generalising from individual studies, certain themes emerge. Barriers to communication presented by the organisation of services, for example the non-availability of professional interpreters at point of need in a general practice, may be exacerbated by gendered provision of service. The apparent double-bind of needing to choose between language or gender matching is an evident concern. If minority ethnic women feel obliged to choose between either using a family member, for example a son, to interpret with a female doctor, or instead seeing a male bilingual doctor of matching ethnicity, the latter might seem preferable for some health concerns (Ahmad et al, 1991, p 331) but then again not for others. The underlying reasons for women's use of particular GPs, including considerations of gender, are under-researched, and the extent to which cultural factors would be invoked by women as explanations is not clear either. All too little research has explored attitudes of male minority ethnic patients to gender issues in consultations with health professionals. Finally there is little research focusing on attitudes of practitioners to gender issues in communicating with minority ethnic patients.

Language, culture and miscommunication

In addition to attitudinal factors in miscommunication, there are also issues connected with aspects of language use and awareness. Problems of miscommunication and language use may influence care and treatment and also contribute to the reinforcement of stereotyping behaviour. These problems may occur when practitioners communicate with minority ethnic patients alone, with family members present, or with professional interpreters or linkworkers. This section focuses on cultural and linguistic difficulties with the use of the same language, before attention is turned to multi-party communication.

Different meanings of words and phrases

One way in which professional practice may contribute to communication barriers is through conflating communication difficulties with a reductive view of the linguistic deficit of patients. In one study of 32 health professionals' views of communication difficulties in Melbourne, Australia, the professionals were far more aware of difficulties arising from lack of a shared language than from cultural and linguistic differences in the use of the same language (Pauwels, 1990, p 99). Viewing communication issues in a limited way can itself then contribute to miscommunication.

Miscommunication might arise from differences in the meaning of words or phrases (lexico-semantic differences), for example in metaphorical expressions of health problems:

"... a chill entered my body."

"I have bad blood." (Pauwels, 1990, p 105)

While practitioners might recognise the cultural provenance of such expressions, the problem remains that similar expressions may have overlapping but distinct connotations across cultures (Pauwels, 1990, p 105). For example, expressions of mental distress may take linguistic forms that suggest a partly culture-specific and partly universal understanding of the relationship between emotion, bodily sensation and thought. In a study of culture and the expression of mental distress, interviews held in Punjabi and Urdu with South Asian women in Bristol elicited instances of the linguistic structuring of thought and feeling like this:

> "... people came to pay their respects ... my heart kept falling.... I felt as if my head was about to burst. I'd tie my head and hold it.... I do all this thinking in my heart ... I know it affects the brain but what can I do? That blow hit me as if my heart had stopped.... I think, think, think in my heart ... this built up pressure in my head...."
> (Fenton and Sadiq Sangster, 1996, p 76)

In translating their perceptions into English, patients may feel that part of the meaning is lost:

> "... you see I can explain myself in English somewhat but I can't tell him how I am feeling – what is in my heart.... I can't get the right words." (Fenton and Sadiq Sangster, 1996, pp 76-8)

These quotes illuminate the intricate relationship between language and socio-culturally sanctioned ways of communicating experience. Clearly such a problem of expression poses challenges to practitioners who 'get by' without identifying communication support needs. A challenge for education is to strengthen practitioners' cognitive understandings of the complexity of patient health experiences and expressions, rather than to generate stereotypes of culturally contrasting health belief systems.

Meanings in context

Another concern is that practitioner awareness of obvious differences in meanings of words or phrases and grammatical differences in expression is not usually matched by awareness of the types of indirect interpersonal communication failure that can occur. For example, in a study of views of doctors, nurses and midwives in Melbourne (Pauwels, 1990), respondents had difficulties in interpreting the reported reluctance of some patients whose first language was not English to answer some open questions like:

"... what can I do for you?"

"... where is the pain?"

as opposed to closed questions such as:

"... the pain is stronger here isn't it?"

Various possibilities are suggested for the minimal responses of patients. Some questions might be difficult to understand grammatically, and a pause might indicate a vocabulary deficit or the time required for non-fluent speakers to produce an answer. Arguably, as well, some open, information-seeking questions might undermine expectations about the role relationship between clinician as 'expert' and patient (Pauwels, 1990, p 107). Also, silences, responsive expressions such as 'mmhmm', and repetitions might be intended primarily to express interpersonal meanings (Brown and Levinson, 1987), like embarrassment, or alternatively to indicate comprehension. Such ambiguities of meaning can contribute to miscommunication.

In sum, an important factor in miscommunication could be the use by professionals of a limiting sense-making framework when attributing meaning to communicative difficulties in intercultural health interactions. If communication strategies adopted by professionals are perceived to fail, this might potentially reinforce culturally stereotyping explanations of problems (Roberts, 1998, p 120).

Language, miscommunication and culture in multi-party communication

Meaning-making processes in face-to-face communication are reliant in part on people's inferential capacities and knowledge frameworks for interpreting talk. These capacities and frameworks are not necessarily perfectly matched between participants. Inferences about intentions can go wrong where there is relatively little history of shared communicative styles, and then the social and emotional intelligence aspects of communication may be as important as the ideational ones (Roberts, 1998, pp 119-22).

In multi-party, transcultural communication between practitioners, patients and their carers, or interpreters, problems may arise through aspects of inaccurate translation and through misunderstandings about participant roles. Studies have shown, for example, that translation may alter information or relationship messages by omission of detail, substitution of one concept for another, conceptual simplification (Farooq et al, 1997, p 211), and addition of information (Hornberger et al, 1996, p 849). With professional translators there is also the loss of confidentiality and the introduction of a potential intermediary influence on decision making (Pauwels, 1990, p 101). An interpreter may have cultural affiliations to lay and/or professional community perspectives, with varying consequences for interaction and understandings (Hatton and Webb, 1993).

Using a family member may present problems through confusion of roles, barriers to patient disclosure in, for example, domestic conflicts, and also unintentional mistranslation. Yet, patients in some situations may prefer to be supported within the interdependent culture of their family than to rely on professional interpreters, as this may raise larger confidentiality concerns and detract from the building of empathy (Gerrish, 2001). However, among the 'cultural mediation' tasks of an intermediary, which may be difficult for family members, is the necessary shifting of roles and languages between the clinical world view and language of medicine, and the everyday world view and language of the user (Hasselkus, 1992, p 301).

Implications of process barriers for practitioners

Practitioner education should perhaps include some basic, introductory awareness raising. An important factor in miscommunication may be the over-attribution by practitioners of problems to grammatical and vocabulary difficulties and the underestimation of pragmatic issues (Pauwels, 1990, p 109; Rehbein, 1994, pp 83-130). This might lead practitioners to adopt insufficient communication strategies for:

- supporting patients in defining their own communication needs;
- raising expectations about upcoming communication events;
- signalling any difficulties or providing opportunities for patients to do so; and
- attending, listening, and retrospectively clarifying understanding about communicative events.

Practitioners clearly need the communication skills to assess users' beliefs and values about health and health care as far as these are relevant to clinical practice. A common issue for the women in a qualitative study of views of 20 Glaswegian South Asian women on communication with their GPs (Bowes and Domokos, 1995a, pp 22-33) was that the GPs were not listening to them properly, instead sometimes complaining that the women were presenting with trivial worries. Also, minority ethnic women may reach decisions about health care using several sources, including community and family resources (Bowes and Domokos, 1995a, p 29).

Of course, communication skills, such as the ability to ask questions and explain health procedures and options in an unrushed and caring manner, still require a foundation in knowledge. For example, areas such as diet, religion and hygiene preferences provide a framework for enquiry, while, on the other hand, some behaviours, questions and words may be offensive, for some people (Shah, 1997, pp 42-3). However, a concern is that knowledge frameworks have sometimes been modelled in an inappropriate way, as static instead of dynamic, with over-generalised ethnic categories; and without due emphasis on the impacts of language processes, of class, age and gender differences, and of biographical experience on individuals' beliefs and concerns. This may then contribute to stereotyping.

The issues concerning stereotyping and racial discrimination need to be addressed more robustly in educational programmes. It might be helpful to encourage practitioners to develop a deeper understanding of the complexities connecting language, the process of stereotyping, and broader structural processes to do with racial discrimination. There are concerns regarding incompatibilities between academic models and theories and theories-in-use (Greenwood, 1993). This issue might be influenced by the socialisation processes that practitioners experience in specific workplace cultures, for example hospital wards and primary care teams. This matter requires addressing in training. Reflective practice modules might encourage practitioners to explore the shaping influence of workplace cultures on individual practice, and to consider strategies to reduce discrepancies.

TWO

Structural barriers

This chapter focuses on several areas where organisational aspects undermine the quality of communication and care. The primary focus of the chapter is on the UK. At a time when DoH-led organisational reforms encourage local community empowerment (DoH, 2001a) and user self-management of health care (DoH, 2001b), it is vital that users should not be excluded due to communication barriers limiting their control over care options. In the areas of assessment of minority ethnic user needs by community consultation, gathering and use of information about individual patients' communication needs, bilingual support, practitioner education, and provision of material resources, organisational shortcomings have been demonstrated.

User needs and access

A starting point, for the development of effective communication, and an equitably resourced service, must be an adequate assessment of user communication needs. In the case of minority ethnic communities, a central factor is the procedures, including user consultation, by which communication needs are assessed. Communication needs are closely related to peoples' beliefs, attitudes, knowledge and past experiences, which influence wants and expectations (Baxter, 1993, p 8). Felt needs, in terms of user attitudes to such issues as privacy, consent and religion, have to be taken into account. Such factors are culture-related and are historically dynamic. For example, refugees and asylum seekers may have experiences shaped by current unemployment levels as high as 100%; depression; and recently survived torture (Stephenson, 1995, p 1631;Trinh, 1996, p 1; Free et al, 1999 p 373) Felt needs are influenced in turn by other changing factors such as linguistic background, age profile, gender, and socio-economic status (Shah and Piracha, 1993, p 40). Communities may be highly differentiated internally, and preferences for a language-matched service may well change over time and with generational shift. For example, among refugees and asylum seekers, some of whom may be traumatised, the need for supportive provision such as advocacy and interpreting services may best be monitored by planning processes that empower community members to assert their own developing requirements (Trinh, 1996, pp 1, 24). Such processes demand creative thinking, inter-agency collaboration, and mobilisation of community-based resources, such as linkworkers. In general, a needs assessment process which ignores user and provider beliefs, knowledge and experiences, is likely to fail (Baxter, 1993, p 8).

Yet development of adequate consultation is itself a challenging process. Some serious attempts have been made to involve community representatives from an early stage (Karim, 1996, p 6). For example, the Riverside Community Health Care Trust set up a Somali linkworker project with certain expectations about user needs, identifying the linkworker herself as the key to accessing previously unanticipated perceptions of need (Shea, 1997, pp 14-15). Lack of bilingual support is a particular barrier to identifying the needs of community members who are not fluent in English, some of whom may also be quite socially isolated and not prominent in community structures.

A review of projects throughout the UK conducted for Buckinghamshire Health Authority (BHA) found that a recurrent barrier to user involvement in needs assessment is the distinction between user views and community gatekeeper views (BHA, 1996, pp 44-6). Community leaders are not the sole representatives of the views of a particular community. However, liaison work is important as their influence may be essential (BHA, 1996, p 45). For example, a degree of personal understanding and experience of linkworker services by community leaders can influence the access of newly arrived women to health facilities (Clevely Northgate Trust, 1987, cited in BHA, p 45).

An approach to consultation about communication needs is recommended that focuses on developing informal and semi-formal links between service developers, practitioners and community members (for example using focus groups or existing community centres) is recommended (BHA, 1996, p 56). Otherwise, services may not be accessed, through ignorance of their existence or uncertainty and misapprehension about their purpose and relevance, and doubts about the roles of health professionals. In addition, users may also have difficulties negotiating a passage through different sectors. There may be problems in developing a responsive service, and, for practitioners, problems in understanding and responding to user requirements.

Lack of user knowledge of availability and range of services

A further problem posing organisational challenges is that services may not be well understood by particular communities, including individuals who are not fluent in English. For example, a qualitative focus group study of access to and use of out-of-hours service by three Vietnamese community groups in South London found that most participants did not know about out-of-hours services, were not aware of emergency appointments, and were unable to use telephones in English for emergency calls (Free et al, 1999, p 369). At the same time, service providers arranged no interpreters outside normal working hours and offered no direct access to interpreters (Free et al, 1999, p 371). A survey of elderly inner city residents of West Birmingham found lower awareness of the existence of all community health services by Asian-born respondents than three other study groups (UK born, 'West Indian' born, and 'Other') (Ritch et al, 1996, p 217). Poor knowledge of services was also a key finding of a qualitative study of the communication needs of pregnant minority ethnic women in Salford (Baxter, 1993, p 3). The examples of refugees, elderly people, and women all present concerns about crossing barriers of English language fluency in information provision.

Principles for resource allocation

Related to the adequacy of consultation mechanisms, sound principles for resource allocation are a further necessary condition underlying the provision of sufficient communication resources to meet the needs of minority ethnic communities. The principle should not be to provide equal resources to all but to adapt health care services to the requirements of culturally diverse populations, to ensure more equal treatment outcomes (Saldov and Chow, 1994, p 126). This equity requires the removal of structural barriers to communication, and the development of culture-sensitive health services (Saldov and Chow, 1994, p 126).
For example, A&E departments may be open to all for 24 hours a day, but unless there is a professional interpreting service available at the point of need for 24 hours a day there can be no equity (Karim, 1996, p 68). Reliance on non-professional interpreters would be inequitable if, for example, a result would be "misdiagnoses, mistreatments, wasted time in the search for effective interpretation, and delays in the course of treatment" (Saldov and Chow, 1994, p 120).

Equity of access to health records and complaints procedures

Two further problems have been identified as obstructing access and participation. First, without adequate bilingual support when necessary, minority ethnic patients do not enjoy equity of access to health records (Arora et al, 1995, p 8). Second, without bilingual support or translated materials when necessary, some minority patients are unlikely to understand health complaints procedures. Both these problems are, of course, related to the process issue that practitioners do not always provide individual users with opportunities to ask questions and state preferences (Small et al, 1999).

The lack of equity is suggested in a survey of patients at a hospital A&E department which showed lower levels of complaining by minority ethnic patients than 'white' patients (Karim, 1996, pp 70-1). The survey also showed that a slightly higher percentage of minority ethnic patients than white patients had wished to complain, and that a slightly higher proportion of minority ethnic patients did not know how to complain. Many patients of all ethnic origins did not know who to direct their complaints to. It is recommended that the complaints procedure should be publicised better, and in different languages (Karim, 1996, p 74). Procedures for making oral complaints need to be made known to those who may not be able to read or write sufficiently in any language (Karim, 1996, p 74; Lawrenson et al, 1998, p 122).

To summarise the access and participation issues raised so far, interrelated problems of communication have been identified that can hinder minority ethnic communities from using services. Issues have been highlighted of:

- consultation with minority ethnic user groups;
- user knowledge of the availability and range of services;
- user opportunity to access linguistically comprehensible services, ask for information, exercise choice, and provide feedback on service quality.

Getting through the system

Once initial contact with health services is made, a further potential problem is the quality of resources that support minority ethnic service users in moving through the system. Among the barriers which have been identified are:

- the organisation of communications at key stages and points of access; and
- quality and use of ethnic monitoring systems to ensure sufficient and appropriate resource provision across the service.

Organisational barriers at points of transition across service stages or sectors

Organisational failure to support culturally appropriate communications may contribute to attrition, frustrate continued access to the various stages of health care, and negate practitioners' efforts. For example, a focus group study of factors deterring non-English-speaking women from cervical screening found high levels of uncertainty about the procedures involved. Some women could not remember receiving call–recall letters, or, without someone to translate, they ignored them; some did not know laboratory analysis was involved; and many were not aware that cervical screening had to be repeated regularly (Naish et al, 1994, p 1126). Recommendations for improving patients' understanding of processes involving repeat visits include:

- provision of bilingual advocates;
- health information leaflets produced by advocates through community consultation (Naish et al, 1994, p 1127).

At the different points of access to health resources, non–provision of bilingual staff, where and where these are wanted, can lead to communication breakdown and attrition. This may occur, for example, where general practitioners never employ professional interpreters, and have no system of formally monitoring ethnicity or communication needs of patients they serve, since this is not mandatory in primary care (Farshi et al, 1999, p 24).

The role of receptionists in enabling or disabling minority ethnic patients from accessing resources has been acknowledged (Arai and Farrow, 1995, p 357). At this stage, not being understood might mean not getting treated, not only in terms of appointment systems, but also in terms of recording relevant information which would be used to identify need throughout the system. For example, a survey of user views of language issues in community health provision in Bradford found that:

- 42% of 241 minority ethnic respondents felt that they could communicate with receptionists only a little or not at all;
- 47% of respondents felt that they could neither read nor understand appointments;
- 66.4% thought bilingual receptionists would be very useful. (Arora et al, 1995, pp 30, 32–4)

In acute care, a result of problems in communication at reception can be delays in retrieving records, in proper registration, and in being called for treatment (Karim, 1996, pp 58–9). Recommendations include:

- developing a system which would encourage patients medical cards to travel with the patients to provide quicker access to information;
- training receptionists in naming systems (Karim, 1996, p 61); ·and
- targeting reception as a priority area for appointment of bilingual workers (Arora et al, 1995, p 42).

Monitoring of ethnicity and communication requirements

A further influence on patients' success or failure in passing through the system and having satisfactory interactions with practitioners may be the systems and categories used to identify ethnicity. A recent study of ethnic monitoring by A&E departments in one regional health authority (North Thames) found problems related to insufficiently systematic data collection, and a lack of clarity about how data would be analysed and used (Lawrenson et al, 1998, pp 117–23); service units recorded data in a way that fits in with the broad categories used in the 1991 census (pp 120–1). This causes problems where, for example, a category like 'Bangladeshi', as opposed to 'Asian', or a category like 'mixed parentage/ dual heritage' is unavailable to those who might wish to use it. It is recommended that choices for ethnic category should be "determined locally", through community consultation, and in relation to the purposes for which data is collected (Lawrenson et al, 1998, p 121; Monach and Davis, 1996, p 11). This implies collection of information relevant to provision of interpreters, and translation of health materials (Monach and Davis, 1996, p 11).

At the same time, patients may be concerned, from past experience, about the use that is made of ethnic data. Issues of trust and confidentiality can be a massive barrier to relationship building. Monitoring, or patient profiling, needs to be carried out sensitively by trained staff, with purposes and categories clarified through community consultation, so that concerns about confidentiality might be alleviated (Monach and Davis, 1996, pp 63–5).

In particular, the absence of ethnic and language monitoring in general practice can cause delays or misunderstandings in provision of needed resources throughout a health care career since referrals from GPs are normally the route to specialist consultations (Monach and Davis, 1996, p 10). Inadequate monitoring also hampers the evaluation and targeting of service provision in relation to expressed health needs (Monach and Davis, 1996, p 11; Arora et al, 1995, p 41). A recording system is needed that makes minimum demands of literacy and English language skills, and which allows, if necessary, for initial storing of information in languages other than English.

To ensure satisfactory patient referrals, appointments procedures need to be developed to ascertain communication requirements (Arora et al, 1995, p 41), while a computerised system might carry this information across the different health sectors (Levenson and Gillam, 1996, p 43; Baxter et al, 1996; Warrier and Goodman, 1996).

Bilingual services

A consequence of inadequate community consultation and ethnic monitoring is that some users' particular needs and preferences for bilingual services will not be recognised, or not recognised at the right time. The lack of bilingual services at the point of need has been documented. For example, in primary care in the UK, GPs and practice nurses' use of interpreters has been minimal (Lam and Green, 1994, pp 293–9; Farshi et al, 1999, p 24). Yet this undermines the principle of equity, reinforced by policy statements such as the DoH's *The vital connection* (2000). Health advocates and linkworkers are relatively scarce, but also have a role to play in facilitating equitable processes (Karim, 1996, p 74; Lawrenson et al, 1998, p 122), for example concerning information, access and referrals (Arora et al, 1995, p 8).

Structural factors that influence the low use of bilingual resources may include booking systems, and funding arrangements. It is suggested that many practitioners are not made aware of the range of available resources, or that access procedures are too complicated (Farshi et al, 1999, pp 26–7). This may be coupled with inadequate professional recognition of interpreters, linkworkers and advocates (Leather et al, 1996, p 5). Not all patients with limited English are made fully aware, for example through translated information sheets, of their rights and opportunities to request professional bilingual support. Underlying such accounts, a central obstacle to the enhancement of bilingual support services may be insufficient acknowledgement, throughout the NHS, of the need.

Yet there is no doubt that bilingual support is high on the priority list of many service users who lack fluency in English. For example, in a survey of 241 users of Bradford Community Health Trust, respondents were asked why they found it difficult to access services. The lack of interpreters was the most frequently cited barrier (Arora et al, 1995, p 37). At the A&E department at Birmingham Heartlands Hospital, 59% of 370 minority ethnic patients did not know that the hospital has a professional interpreting service (Karim, 1996, p 62). While some may see advantages in using relatives and friends to interpret, patients should be fully aware of their rights and opportunities for professional bilingual support.

Organisation of bilingual services

Major barriers to communication have been found in the organisation of bilingual services. Most linkworker and advocacy posts have been provided through short-term funding and this restricts the development of a community's access to services, limits the embedding of services within the NHS, and blights the careers and employment prospects of the workers (Levenson and Gillam, 1998, p 32). Bilingual workers are often employed on short term contracts and low salary levels, which may damage their status (Levenson and Gillam, 1998, pp 34-5; Baxter et al, 1996, p 14). Such issues can dent morale and lead to resignations (Rocheron et al, 1989, 71).

Problems have been identified arising from the lack of an effective and responsive management structure for bilingual services. For example, an Australian study of community mental health services found that few bilingual staff had access to any mechanisms for raising concerns or participating in service development (Mitchell et al, 1998, p 431). Difficulties sometimes arise when linkworkers lack minority ethnic representation in their management structures (Rocheron et al, 1989a, pp 121-2) or lack a mentor (Shea, 1997, p 17). Many linkworkers see their role drawing strength from their community links. Yet this is made difficult if the role lacks all autonomy from nursing establishments, and if consultations on role development between the health service and community groups and voluntary organisations are inadequate (Rocheron et al, 1989a, p 120; Levenson and Gillam, 1998, p 41).

It has been recommended that bilingual services require a management structure independent of clinical management structures (Baxter et al, 1996, p 9; Levenson and Gillam, 1998, p 41), and require active support from line managers and senior management. Without this support it is difficult for bilingual staff to advocate changes in existing practices, or to challenge the racism which has been noted in several reports (Rocheron et al, 1989a, p 124; Chahal, 1996, p 68). In general, bilingual services have been impeded through lack of feedback mechanisms and problems of line management and accountability.

Training of bilingual health workers

While advocates and linkworkers draw strength from experience within a minority ethnic community, experience is no substitute for training when it comes to some core knowledge and skill requirements, such as health service and medical knowledge, interpreting skills, administrative skills, and professional standards (Leather et al, 1996, p 10).

Further, it is arguable that, without adequate training, the tensions implicit in the advocacy role, which involves supporting and advising clients and also advising professionals, might be unmanageable, especially in a context requiring awareness of equal opportunities, racism and prejudice (Bahl, 1988, p 10). Yet, despite the need, initial and subsequent training of bilingual workers varies widely in length and content among agencies (Baxter et al, 1996, p 14). The lack of nationally accredited courses for linkworkers has probably contributed to their low status among health staff (Levenson and Gillam, 1998, p 39; Podro, 1994).

It has also been argued that training bilingual staff without training other health service professionals is inadequate (Baxter et al, 1996, p 4; Gerrish, 2001). However, no published evaluations of such training involving other professionals were uncovered for this report, nor in an earlier report (Levenson and Gillam, 1998, p 39).

Employment profile mechanisms and issues around resource targeting

A problem for trained bilingual staff is that poor ethnic monitoring of patients and of staff and a poor system of consultation with service users about needs leads to underemployment. The Language Needs Assessment project survey of services provided by Bradford Community Health Trust concluded that managers should develop service take-up profiles by ethnic origin and match these with employee profiles to target areas for bilingual recruitment (Arora et al, 1995, p 42).

This was not being done – of 35 managers interviewed only 11.4% systematically identified the language needs of the user (Arora et al, 1995, p 20).

The problematic issue of matching staff with user language is related to the issue of the distribution of bilingual staff throughout the health service. The low representation of minority ethnic staff in senior posts is a specific concern (Bhatt and Dickinson, 1993, p 92).

In situations of identified need for bilingual workers, distribution of work between linkworkers and interpreters may also be an issue, especially in community settings. Where services are not known about or well understood, there may be a need for advocates and linkworkers (as opposed to interpreters only) in health promotion roles, who empathise with a community's needs and perceptions and who can also educate health workers as well as community members (Baxter et al, 1996, pp 5, 18).

There may be a need for greater involvement of bilingual workers with carers of older people, people with chronic illness, or people with disabilities from non–English-speaking backgrounds in the home. The relatively low uptake of full-time residential care by minority ethnic communities does not mean that families 'look after their own' without difficulties and have no need or wish for culturally sensitive and, where appropriate, bilingual support services (Plunkett and Quine, 1996, pp 28-9; Hatton et al, 1998, pp 821-37).

It is important to identify the cultural resources within community and families which carers draw on in assessing the meaning and value of services. Bilingual staff, for example interpreters, should be "trained and experienced in interpreting between professionals and *families*", while "a thorough understanding of the terms used by professionals and an empathic approach to families are essential" (Hatton et al, 1998, p 834; author's italics).

Overall, therefore, the implementation of much-needed bilingual support has to be responsive to the concerns of user communities. More generally the recruitment, training and deployment of bilingual workers has to be coordinated strategically in response to clear goals and principles.

Material resources and media

Shortcomings of consultation, and culturally sensitive assessment of patient needs may contribute to a further barrier to participation – insufficient or inappropriate use of information materials and media.

Some identified concerns with the use of materials and media include:

- the language of resources, that is, untranslated materials;
- the quality of translated and untranslated materials;
- the lack of appropriate variety of information resources.

Translation

Problems have been identified with the insufficient quantity of appropriately translated information. For example, the Language Needs Assessment project survey of 120 minority ethnic users and 35 managers of Bradford Community Health Trust found that 73% of users preferred health information to be in the appropriate Asian languages, yet only 17% of managers provided information in languages other than English (Arora et al, 1995, p 39).

The situation is complicated by the fact that some studies have found that a high proportion of the patients who cannot read materials in English also cannot read them in the appropriate community written language (Arora et al, 1995, p 30; Karim, 1996, p 45). The issue of whether translated information will actually be read needs to be considered in the light of research into the population to be served (Karim, 1996, p 50).

Translating material into one or two community languages may also leave some minority ethnic patients unable to read information because they cannot read in those languages. Chinese communities, for example, may be less well served than South Asian communities who read Urdu (Baxter et al, 1996, p 15; Bhatt and Dickinson, 1993, p 82). Targeting users who under-utilise services, for example older people, increases the likelihood that translation alone (without the use of other media and /or personal contacts) would prove insufficient.

Quality of materials

A related issue is the quality of written information. If materials are produced without sufficient consultation and attention to audience and purpose, readability suffers. For example, a study of views of minority ethnic women about cervical screening found that the translated information leaflets presupposed familiarity with the NHS and an interest in cervical smears, which for many was an unfamiliar topic (Box, 1998, p 9). Issues of clarity, layout, translation quality and culturally competent content should be ascertained through community consultations and pre-testing (Shea, 1997, p 6).

Variety of information resources

A major barrier to effective use of material resources would appear to be the insufficient use of an appropriate variety of resources. There appears to be under-utilisation of audio-visual resources for health information compared to translated leaflets (Arora et al, 1995, p 36-9); a national survey involving 277 members of seven different language groups found a common preference for video over all other media among South Asian and Chinese respondents (Bhatt and Dickinson, 1993, p 86). Several studies recommend the use of videotapes, to complement written information (Shah, 1993, p 41; Karim, 1996, p 104). The Bradford CHT study recommends that audio-visual material should be promoted through outreach work in community centres, homes and health centres (Arora et al, 1995, p 43).

Another issue concerns the possible use of pictorial signs. It has been argued that pictorial representations should be combined with linguistic signs in hospitals and health centres, since linguistic information may not be understood by all users even when it is translated (Karim, 1996, p 51).

Problems in understanding and recalling medication instructions or health information leaflets are obviously a serious barrier to patient compliance and health, especially when functional literacy is an issue. Such problems might be widespread especially among the elderly. One approach that has been advocated is the use of pictograms in pharmacy practice (Dowse and Ehlers, 1998, p 109). Studies with literate populations suggest that pictograms, when used alone, are not very effective, but with textual material or person-to-person communication they may prove effective in enhancing comprehension and ultimately compliance (Dowse and Ehlers, 1998, p 111).

Professional training and communication practice

While there is emerging evidence that practitioner education in transcultural communication can enhance practice, much remains to be understood about the mechanisms and contexts through which educational programmes can be implemented effectively (Gerrish et al, 1996).

There is some evidence that without specialised training, experience does not equip practitioners with all the skills, awareness and knowledge to achieve culturally competent communication. A questionnaire survey of 191 palliative care practitioners in Perth, Australia, found no significant association between the total time spent working in palliative care and the practitioners' self-perceived competence for scenarios with minority ethnic groups, but a significant association between specific training and experience (McNamara et al, 1997, p 363). Similarly, a questionnaire survey of 68 physiotherapists in two UK health authorities found that although contact with Bangladeshi people increased perceived awareness of their culture, this did not result in fewer perceived problems with physiotherapy management (Jaggi and Bithell, 1995, p 330).

Educational courses are needed to support practitioners in the long-term process of acquiring transcultural communication competence. McNamara et al recommend that educational programmes for transcultural communication should include:

- language guidelines for working across boundaries;
- information regarding access to specific communication resources;
- strategies for dealing with constraints in using bilingual services for example constraints of access;
- professional practice with bilingual professionals;
- knowledge of cultural beliefs and practices; and
- workshops on ethical cross-cultural decision-making. (McNamara et al, 1997, pp 365-6)

Even within this useful, but rather functional and individualistic list, obvious elements are missing, for example adapting, for users who are not fluent in English, aspects of interpersonal skills such as:

- Developing care plans with users which address needs for language help.
- Supportive discussion of preferences for care. (Small et al, 1999, p 97)

There is also an absence of focus on the structural aspects of racism, institutional organisation and culture. A problem may be that the teaching of interpersonal communication skills is not effectively integrated within a broader transcultural competence framework. A survey of common foundation programme curricula for nursing and midwifery pre-registration training across the UK evaluated courses for the extent to which they include topics such as:

- concepts of ethnicity, culture and race;
- minority ethnic health needs;
- minority ethnic access to services;
- legislative implications for health care provision;
- culturally appropriate assessment and identification of need; and
- intercultural communication. (Gerrish et al, 1996, p 57)

What remains to be explored is a range of educational strategies for integrating communication in the broad sense outlined in this book with the other curricular components.

Organisational barriers to training implementation

While almost no work has been published evaluating in-service courses, barriers to effectiveness in the training of pre-registration nurses and midwives have been illuminated in a qualitative study combining a national survey with detailed interview and observational data from three specific educational institutions (Gerrish et al, 1996).

Problems are identified in course curricula, in practice settings, and in the recruitment of minority ethnic trainees. Few programmes made it a formal requirement for students to confront concepts of ethnicity and race, and intercultural communication (Gerrish et al, 1996, p 56). There were apparent problems of divisional coordination, and managerial inertia was partly blamed for this (p 65). Practice placements were not consistently arranged in areas of ethnic diversity (p 71). In practice settings, trainees sometimes lacked adequate mentoring when they encountered instances of resource shortages, and also of racist behaviour from professionals (p 81).

The training and employment of more minority ethnic practitioners is widely viewed as a necessary step to improving communication with minority ethnic users of health services. Yet the reasons why different minority ethnic communities are under-represented in the health service professions may be as much to do with perceptions of institutional racism and unattractive conditions as with cultural sanctions on specific caring roles (Gerrish et al, 1996, p 109).

Implications for health practitioners

This chapter has discussed structural and organisational barriers to communication, focusing on community consultation mechanisms, monitoring and use of information about patients' communication needs, the provision of bilingual resources, and organisation of training. Organisational shortcomings impede communication between individuals, and increase the pressure on practitioners to communicate with exceptional competence. It may be argued that the competence of practitioners in health care teams depends in part on their ability to identify organisational conditions that enhance rather than stifle transcultural interaction. Practitioner education should perhaps encourage practitioners to reflect on communication competencies in key areas, both at individual and organisational levels.

Conclusions

The last two chapters have indicated that barriers to communication persist at interpersonal, organisational, and cultural levels. It is suggested that the enhancement of communication depends on recognising relationships between these levels, and on developing appropriate, context-sensitive strategies for change.

This chapter has indicated how organisational influences encourage or deter effective community consultation, ethnic monitoring, and use of bilingual and material resources. Inadequate user consultation can lead to provision of services which are not well understood by those who would use them, and not well adapted to meet the users' needs. Barriers have also been identified in systems for collecting and using information about minority ethnic patients' linguistic and cultural needs.

There are also problems of communicating health information to minority ethnic clients in effective, targeted ways.

The organisation of bilingual services remains inadequate, in terms of recruitment and training, deployment, management, and negotiation of roles. Another area where barriers persist is that of insufficient or inappropriate use of material resources for health education and information.

A final area where structural barriers impact on the quality of communication processes is the training of health professionals. There is a need for further research on the effectiveness of existing transcultural and anti-racist communication training, especially at an in-service or post-registration level, taking into account delivery mechanisms, practice contexts, and outcomes.

A key concern in turning from the discussion of barriers to the review of interventions which follows will be how communication processes are conceptualised. The barriers research indicates numerous links between structural problems and processes of 'miscommunication'. The barrier studies also clarify aspects of the qualities of transcultural communication processes. Important issues raised here for the evaluation of interventions are:

> … if and how they generate insights into transcultural communication processes, viewed in terms of quality assurance as well as in terms of the impact of a 'communication' treatment on important measures of health or health service outcome

and

> … if and how they engage with any significant structural and organisational issues in relation to interpersonal communication processes.

Part two:
Intervention studies

Introduction

The intervention studies reviewed in the next three chapters cover a wide range of communication areas but in a piecemeal way. Some studies are focused at structural and organisational levels. These include an evaluation of external audit as an agent of change in ethnically sensitive primary practice; an evaluations of bilingual services in mental health; an evaluation of an interpreter training project; and an evaluation of an innovation in ethnic monitoring. At the cusp of structural organisation and communication processes are intervention studies examining the impact of bilingual services involving health advocates, or interpreters, or linkworkers on a range of outcome measures. A further group of impact studies focuses on training interventions with clinical professionals, receptionists, and researchers from minority ethnic communities. Other studies concentrate on the impact of specific health communication 'packages' on communities' or individuals' beliefs, knowledge or behaviour. A pair of studies evaluates health education course interventions. A further group of health information impact studies examines different combinations of 'culturally sensitive' media and person-to-person contact interventions.

The majority, but not all, of the intervention studies reviewed here follow a quasi-experimental methodology. The review draws attention to gains and losses in the scope and types of evidence garnered through the chosen methodological approach. Each paper is reviewed using the same descriptive and evaluative format. A number of descriptive entries lead from the 'subject', 'aims', 'methods' and 'rationale' of the study to the 'outcome measures' and 'results'. The authors' discussion of findings is then summarised under the heading 'interpretations'.

An evaluative commentary on the methodology and findings appears under the heading 'evaluation'. Key considerations are whether the study has a method well matched to clear aims, and whether the design and data analysis lead to credibility. A further evaluation of the clarity and adequacy of the authors' discussion appears under the heading 'evaluation of interpretation'. Thematic issues and connections between the studies in upcoming sections are developed under the heading 'themes'. Links between studies that have already been reviewed are highlighted in the sections 'comparisons between studies'. In support of these chapters, Appendix 4 contains tables highlighting some of the key comparisons made in the review between those studies that proved closely comparable. A discussion of key issues arising from the interventions is provided in the final chapter.

THREE

Intervention studies: service development

Evaluation of service organisation: themes

The first study reviewed below is unusual with its explicit focus on overall service organisation and staff practice as the central level of analysis, although studies of specialist services, linkworkers, and interpreters which are reviewed in later sections also focus in some detail on organisational issues. The focus in the first study on auditing organisation and 'ethnically sensitive' practice in selected primary and secondary settings is interesting for two reasons. First, the study conceives service evaluation as an instrument of change, whereas most other studies are concerned to evaluate specific innovations. Second, the study highlights tensions between the culture of change agents and practice organisational culture, without fully working through those tensions.

Study 1

'Using external audit to review ethnically sensitive practice' and 'Analysis of the external audit on ethnically sensitive practice' (Bhatti-Sinclair and Wheal, 1998a, 1998b).

Subject

The intervention developed a tool for conducting external audit, conducted an external audit of ethnically sensitive practice in selected health settings, and evaluated the tool in terms of its effects in implementing changes in communication and other aspects of service development.

Aims

The general aim of the project was to develop an audit tool and review ethnically sensitive policy and practice in selected primary and secondary healthcare settings. Specifically, the project aimed to compare staff and patient views on service quality for black and ethnic minority patients. It also aimed: to provide guidance to staff on improving practice; to make training opportunities available; to identify ways of improving service quality; and to provide feedback.

Rationale

The regional health authority funded the ethnically sensitive practice team to develop the project in the context of regional concern about service responses to needs of minority ethnic communities. The UK Commission for Racial Equality's Race Relations Code of Practice in Primary Health Care provided guidance which, the report alleges, was widely ignored by health authorities. Despite the 1976 Race Relations Act, the 1990 NHS and Community Care Act and the 1991 Patient's Charter, strategic guidance on policy and practice is still needed. Issues such as access, training and communication are not systematically addressed.

Methodology

An external qualitative review used face-to-face in-depth interviews. Two UK hospital departments were chosen and four surgeries agreed to take part from an area where 19.6% of the population are from minority ethnic groups. A five-stage audit cycle was developed.
   The five planned stages of the audit cycle were:

1. Select topic and define content of ethnically sensitive policy and practice
2. Identify standards
3. Conduct observations and interviews
4. Identify changes to be made, produce recommendations, present reports to participating sites
5. Re-audit.

However, stage 5 of the audit cycle was not implemented.

Intervention details

The three chosen areas of focus at stage 1 were:

- implementation of policies and equal opportunities legislation;
- relevance of services;
- knowledge of religious cultural and social needs of black and ethnic minority groups.

Standards devised at stage 2 included: patient access to documentation; impact of communication systems; record-keeping; and availability of specialist services. For staff, standards focused on quality; training levels; skills in working with minority ethnic patients; and knowledge on communication issues.

At stage 3, face-to-face interviews using semi-structured questionnnaires were conducted with 157 respondents (37 patients and 120 staff).

At stage 4 the reports containing site-specific feedback and recommendations were presented to each site. However, the recommendations were received "cautiously" or "as an external attack" except by one site, and this was one reason why the planned re-audit did not occur.

Participants, dates and setting

The external audit was devised and conducted by two "social work academics". Of the 37 patients interviewed, 21 were of "Asian origin"[1], although no further ethnic breakdown is made. No details are given of the patients' age or gender. The 91 staff interviewed on policy and practice included doctors, nurses, health visitors, receptionists and porters, of whom 82 were of "white British origin", and nine of "black British, Asian, Indian, Chinese and black African and Caribbean origin". Directly after a consultation, 29 staff were interviewed.

Outcome measures

The measures of the effectiveness of external audit as an instrument of change would have been applied at stage 5 (the re-audit). The standards devised at stage 2 would have been applied to the re-audit. Instead of stage 5 occurring, sites were offered individualised training and encouraged to undertake internal re-audit.

Results

The audit resulted in a range of findings about current policy and practice. However, without a re-audit the evaluation of the audit tool as an agent of change lacks positive evidence.

Measures of staff policy and practice: of 91 staff interviewed only 36 were familiar with the Patients' Charter; 23 were familiar with equal opportunities policies, but 76% had had no equal opportunities training. Although five of the sites subscribed to the Language Line telephone interpreting service only one person interviewed had used it.

Only three of 37 patients expressed concern about communication with clinical staff, but eight said they were concerned about communication with reception staff. Reception staff had not been prioritised by management for training. Record-keeping systems were inconsistent, and ethnic monitoring systems were not in place.

Interpretations

The authors claim (in spite of the fact that without external re-audit there was no evidence of the impact of audit on ethnically sensitive practice) that the audit cycle worked well overall. It is stated that the cycle up to stage 4 resulted in the majority of sites using the feedback for awareness raising and staff training. Two surgeries reviewed their reception systems and record-keeping systems.

The process of external audit was problematic. Management were not forthcoming about the complexities of managerial accountability. There were problems of consent by more senior staff without full consultations with less senior staff.

External medical audit is uncommon, especially by social work academics, and using qualitative methods. The topic of anti-racist practice is challenging, and the process could be perceived as threatening. However, external audit can potentially provide detachment and creativity. Collaboration between health and social services is also increasingly important, for example in community care. But auditing is difficult if there is a "fundamental conceptual mismatch" between the auditors and those being audited.

The audit cycle, especially if it is repeated regularly, can be used to develop good practice systematically. However, health staff criticised the project severely as they felt excluded from ownership. The audit team lacked status and their credibility was challenged.

The audit process effectively showed that health services provided to the minority ethnic communities were perceived as of a lower standard that those offered to the majority population. Authorities were not providing focused guidance on practice to staff.

Evaluation

The audit cycles stages appear to match the project aims. However, there are problems with the lack of detail about participants (for example, gender and ages) and the lack of any detailed data from the interviews. Methods of data analysis are not explained and the representation of professional views may be heavily filtered. There is no evidence of bias, yet many health professionals rejected the findings.

Evaluation of interpretation

The details of the report do not corroborate its claim that the external audit cycle is effective in leading to improved practice standards. Re-audit was never conducted partly due to staff hostility. But the report illuminates issues that face any research programme investigating communication within a specific health service organisational culture. Problems of status and ownership are explicitly discussed. This raises the question of whether evaluation might better have involved partnership in reaching agreed goals. There is evidently a need for effective interpersonal skills by external auditors or researchers in evaluating sensitive issues.

There is potential in using external audit as an instrument of change in ethnically sensitive communication policy and practice, but the potential advantages of detachment, cross-service comparison, and dialogue, need to be balanced by an ongoing inclusiveness that seeks to involve all stakeholders as far as possible in self-assessment. Without this, it seems likely that the part played by professional and organisational cultures in attitude formation will be left unclarified. Even then the confrontational aspect of asking whether practice is ethnically sensitive or discriminatory is likely to arouse inevitable resistances.

Ethnic monitoring: themes

An important aspect of ethnically sensitive service development is the gathering and use of information about healthcare users' care needs in terms of communication, ethnicity, and culture. This information should then be used as a means of improving resource provision. Ethnic monitoring is mandatory in secondary in-patient but not in primary care, where it has been haphazard. The next study concerns the development of an ethnic monitoring system in primary care.

Study 2

'Primary care ethnic monitoring pilot project' (Monach and Davis, 1996).

Subject

The study reports on a pilot project to introduce a system of ethnic monitoring in primary care.

Aims

The project aimed to establish and evaluate a mechanism that GP practices could use for monitoring the ethnicity, written and spoken language, religion and diet of patients. The project would develop a system for linking information to patients' records, ensure that patients would be asked only once, and train practice staff.

Rationale

GPs are the main entry point to the health service. The introduction of ethnic monitoring in primary practice would allow information on patients' ethnicity, language, diet and religion to follow the patient through the service. Poor monitoring impedes purchasers and providers from measuring uptake rates and ensuring that services are adequate, appropriate and accessible to patients.

Methodology

An advisory group included different stakeholders, and meetings were held with individuals from community groups. A questionnaire and an information leaflet were devised. These were distributed around selected practices and completed questionnaires collected two weeks after the pilot started and then every week. Four practices with significant proportions of minority ethnic patients were selected and one with a predominantly white list. Staff in these practices were trained. A practice staff questionnaire was distributed for completion at the end of the pilot period.

Intervention details

Practice staff were trained, for one or two hours, on ethnicity, classification details, handling patients' responses and questions, and the rationale for monitoring. The forms and information leaflet were translated into languages estimated to be used by practice patients: Arabic, Bengali, Chinese, Somali, Urdu, and Vietnamese. Of a total of 6,609 forms distributed to practices, 3,153 were completed and analysed. Of these, 60 were completed in Urdu and 10 in Arabic and were translated into English.

Extensive consultation on wording, layout and translation of leaflets was carried out with the Advisory Group and minority ethnic group representatives. The data collection was carried out for between 4 and 13 weeks.

Nine of the original 11 targeted practices refused to take part. A further three practices were then targeted. Information systems were so different between practices that it was decided to leave individual practices to devise their own tagging system for preventing duplication of ethnic monitoring with a particular patient. Only three practices did so.

Participants, dates and setting

The study was conducted in five primary care practices in Sheffield, UK, between December 1995 and January 1996. The monitoring was conducted by reception staff and GPs.

Outcome measures

A questionnaire was filled in by staff to supplement the questionnaire data used for ethnic monitoring. The pilot study does not measure the impact of ethnic monitoring on service organisation.

Results

The study successfully monitored 3,125 patients for language, ethnicity, diet, and religion in the five practices. Over 99% of patients completed the forms, 85% of practice staff reported no patient resistance and 100% felt that the system was "workable". The questionnaire and explanatory leaflet were viewed as effective, and translatable. Re-translation of forms would be easier if there were more pre-coded answers. Practices were able to record the data on computer and manual records. The system costs extra staff time.

Liaison and trust with community groups, and the support of the practice team proved very important. The ethnic monitoring system provided vital information for establishing the level of need for such resources as screening, interpreters, translated materials, and dietary and faith requirements.

Interpretations

The authors state the problem that different approaches may be used to define ethnicity. The need to provide a sufficient number of questionnaire options for self-definition is recognised. In Sheffield the pilot study used options for the following ethnic groups: Pakistani, African-Caribbean, Bangladeshi, Yemeni, Chinese, Somali, and mixed parentage. Any ethnic monitoring programme needs to consider the sensitivity of the issues, and to ensure that minority ethnic groups are persuaded that data will be used for their benefit. Planning needs to be locally responsive, and inclusive of all minority ethnic groups including the less visible ones.

The pilot study showed that categories excluded from the 1991 census such as mixed parentage and Yemeni were useful. The evidence overall suggests that the method of collecting data was successful. Yet in secondary care a different system is used, many staff are untrained, and dissatisfaction is rife.

Routine monitoring of language needs can support provision of interpreter services, and videotapes. But attention has to be paid to the sensitivity of requesting information about literacy.

Overall the lessons learned were: the data collection instrument was effective, but adequate resources, extra administration time, and support of practice managers, GPs, and receptionists are crucial. Interpreters may also be needed. Feeding back results to minority ethnic communities can empower them, but concerns about confidentiality needed to be addressed carefully.

Evaluation

The pilot intervention method of measuring quantities of monitored people from different ethnic groups, and practice staff satisfaction with the process, is appropriate to the aim of evaluating the process of recording information. But the objective of developing a tagging system ensuring that patients will only be asked questions once is not met. The training is also not evaluated.

Evaluation of interpretation

The report provides numerous qualitative insights for establishing a monitoring system. However, some problems, including producing a questionnaire which can support rational service development and yet also meet users' self-definitions of ethnicity and need, are not sufficiently considered. The study does not deal with what happens to the information once it has been recorded. This is typical of several pilot projects. The process of ensuring that information is attached to records requires investigation, while the development of systems for use of this information across different care sectors is not considered. Therefore there is no measure of any impact of ethnic monitoring in primary health care on the health service and on patients' lives.

Bilingual services: service matching – thomas

The development of an ethnically sensitive service involves many facets. One possible aspect of this is the use of ethnic monitoring data to ensure human and material resources are matched to clients' communication needs. A distinction is made between matching individual health professionals with clients by language or ethnicity, and developing a service that is specialised because of features such as recruitment and training of culturally and linguistically knowledgeable staff, community ties, and targeted policy and practice development. An example of specialised service development is the provision of mental health services for specific minority ethnic communities or for refugees. The next two studies evaluate aspects of specialist service development, and raise important issues for equity across the health service.

Study 3

'Satisfaction of Vietnamese patients and their families with refugee and mainstream mental health services' (Silove et al, 1997)

Subject

The study examines satisfaction with different mental health services among Vietnamese psychiatric patients. It also identifies important communication variables in the extent of information provided and the ease of negotiating changes of treatment.

Aims

The comparative study aims to assess mental health service satisfaction levels of psychiatric patients from a Vietnamese refugee community and their relatives, in Australia. The study compares specialist services that are targeted to their ethnic group with mainstream services. The study also aims to identify which aspects of specialist services, if any, are considered to be superior to the mainstream services.

Rationale

Members of refugee communities tend to be traumatised and to under-utilise mental health services. Possible deterrents include stigma associated with mental illness, unfamiliarity with services, and preference for traditional healing. Also, communication difficulties, mismatching expectations of treatment plans, and cultural variations in conceptualising illness may present barriers. There is concern that mainstream services may lack cultural sensitivity. Few studies have explored levels of satisfaction with services.

Methodology

Eligible patients were identified retrospectively from records. The services under review were the in-patient units of two general hospitals, community health centres, and specialised refugee mental health services. Treatment satisfaction measures were taken for the centre where the patient had most recently been treated. Consenting patients and one relative were given a questionnaire and a semi-structured interview.

Intervention details

Respondents were informed that the survey aimed to evaluate aspects of the services, including their satisfaction levels.

Participants, dates and setting

Patients born in Vietnam who had received treatment in Liverpool, New South Wales, over a 12-month period between 1992 and 1993 were eligible. Of these 143, 86 (60.1%) took part, as well as 56 relatives who agreed to participate. Of the sample, 52 were men (60.5%). In total, 48 subjects (56%) had last attended the specialist service. None of the subjects who attended the specialised service had been treated in mainstream services, or vice-versa. Of the specialised service patients, 80% had received a diagnosis of anxiety-depression. All the patients treated in community centres and 57% of hospital patients had received a diagnosis of psychotic disorder.

Outcome measures

Home visits were used to administer questionnaires on satisfaction with the services.

An eight–item measure was developed in Vietnamese. The items covered were:

- ease of obtaining help from the service;
- level of satisfaction with treatments;
- perceived usefulness of treatments;
- extent to which trust was established with the therapist;
- ease of communication with members of staff;
- quality of care received;
- extent of information offered;
- ease of negotiating changes in treatment.

Results

Questionnaire measures of satisfaction with services: patients in specialised services were significantly more satisfied with the extent of information offered and the ease of changing treatment programme. They were also marginally more satisfied in ease of obtaining help, quality of communication, and quality of care. Relatives of patients in the specialised services also expressed greater satisfaction with services.

Multiple regression analysis showed that low English fluency and the specialised refugee services accounted for differential ratings.

Semi-structured interview: four out of ten inquiries showed significantly greater satisfaction from specialised refugee service patients. These were:

- extent to which programmes were explained;
- whether the diagnosis was communicated directly;
- whether the diagnosis was explained fully;
- ease of understanding instructions about medications.

Interpretations

The authors state that, among the study limitations, using Vietnamese researchers to evaluate specialist services may generate social desirability effects, especially among the patients with lower English fluency who were less acculturated. But these were equally distributed between both services. The absence of an Australian-born comparison group was a limitation.

The study data confirms that communication processes are factors in levels of satisfaction. Socio-economic and diagnostic variables had little impact on satisfaction. Reasons can only be inferred for the greater satisfaction with the specialist services concerning communication. Among the reasons might be:

- the use of a bicultural counsellor model by the specialist service;
- differences in motivation and expectations;
- differences in the physical environment;
- greater stigma levels of attending mainstream services;
- a possible trend to be more satisfied with an innovative service.

Evaluation

The study aims of comparing levels of service satisfaction seem matched by measures of treatment satisfaction and communication quality. However, a problem is that the high percentage of patients diagnosed with a psychotic disorder in mainstream services contrasts with the high percentage diagnosed with anxiety-depression in the specialised service. The issue of the impact of different clinical disturbances on communication processes is troubling.

Evaluation of interpretation

By using interviews with family members as well as the patients, the study takes into account the importance of continuing care and of family understandings of mental health services. Greater satisfaction with specialist services is attributed to factors involving intercultural mediation such as how information was explained and how diagnoses were communicated. This is highly relevant with current concerns over provision of services for refugees and asylum seekers. However, the study provides little descriptive detail and generates no evidence to support speculation about why services are viewed as effective, compared to a mainstream counterpart. Each of the possible explanations given requires further qualitative research. In the absence of contextual detail about the linguistic and cultural variables, for example what 'bicultural counselling' would mean (if not simply ethnic or linguistic matching), the findings are not transferable.

Yet the study raises important issues, with a scope beyond mental health, concerning 'institutional' communication, and the development of services which are transculturally communicatively competent to meet the needs of specific groups of minority ethnic health care users. A point of interest is the distinction between ethnic or language matching between individuals and service adaptation. In either case, the implementation of an inter-culturally appropriate service requires effective user involvement and organisational collation of ethnic and language information concerning user needs.

Study 4

'Emergency care avoidance: ethnic matching and participation in minority-serving programmes' (Snowden et al, 1995)

Subject

The study examines the impact of mental health service programmes involving the use of ethnic and language matching between client and clinician on the frequency of emergency service use. The impact of ethnic and language matching is also compared with the impact of the client's programme and the extent to which it was 'minority oriented'.

Aims

The study aimed to evaluate ethnic matching and language matching in relationship to mental health service utilisation, and to focus on the use of emergency care as an indicator of client improvement.

Rationale

Ethnic matching has been widely recommended in mental health services in the US but there is a need for robust evidence. The study takes the low use of emergency care as an indirect indicator of client improvement. Emergency care episodes signal failure of treatment to meet client needs. The study also expands the focus beyond interpersonal client–clinician relationships to include comparison of minority-serving programmes with mainstream ones.

Methodology

The study was conducted in an ethnically diverse county in California, US. Data were taken from the county management records, which show all service use including emergency care in public programmes. All clients receiving outpatient mental health services during fiscal years 1987-88 and 1989-90 were included. A variable was constructed to represent the proportion of "non-white" clients in each programme. The programme level variable was used to indicate the extent to which the proportion of minority presence in a client's programme explained his or her level of emergency service. Minority clients were also classified according to whether they were seen in an ethnically matched relationship, a language-matched relationship, an ethnically and language-matched relationship, or in none. 'Regression analysis' was used to examine relationships between ethnic matching and emergency care use among African-American, Hispanic and Asian clients, between language matching and emergency care use among Hispanic and Asian clients, and between ethnic matching combined with language matching and emergency care use.

Intervention details

Independent variables categorised in the study were gender, ethnicity (contrasted with "white"), age, education, employment status, therapist gender, therapist status, minority ethnic language match, and therapist ethnicity match. The number of emergency visits during the year after an initial outpatient episode was the dependent variable.

Participants, dates and setting

All clients were included who received outpatient mental health services from the selected county's funded programmes during the fiscal years 1987-88 and 1989-90. Approximately 66% were white, 16% were Hispanic, 9% were Asian, and 9% were black. Most clients were aged 25-44, unmarried and unemployed. Around 55% were male.

Outcome measures

Measures of frequency of use of emergency services were associated with patient–professional relationship by ethnic match and by language match, and with match of patient ethnicity to type of mental health service.

Results

Measures of patterns of use of service: participation in an ethnically matched relationship by blacks, Hispanics and Asians was significantly associated with reduced emergency visits by .09 visits per year.

- Participation in a language matched relationship by Hispanics and Asians was also significantly associated with reduced emergency visits by .085 visits per year.
- Participation in a relationship that was both ethnically matched and language matched was significantly associated with reduced emergency visits by .11 visits.
- Clients participating in a minority-serving programme made .04 fewer visits in one year and .01 fewer visits in the second year for every 10% increase in the proportion of minority clients in the programme.

Interpretations

The authors state that ethnic and language matching were associated with lower levels of use of emergency services. This implies avoidance by clients of major crises or coping by alternative means. Yet participation in a minority-serving programme was an equally important predictor of reduced use of emergency services.

As the proportion of minority clients on a programme increases, the norms of interaction and clinical practice on the programme change to reflect the cultural style of the specific minority group in question. But the proportion of minority clients on a programme is only a proxy measure for identifying minority-serving programmes. Such programmes are defined by organisational and clinical features, including:

- recruitment and training of culturally knowledgeable staff;
- culturally sensitive clinical practice;

- developing community ties;
- developing appropriate programme policies.

Such features need to be identified empirically.

Evaluation

In addition to the stated study aim of evaluating ethnic matching and language matching, a further major aim emerges in the report of evaluating minority services in relationship to emergency service use. This addition and the subsequent proxy definition of the minority service create a certain lack of focus in the report, though not the study. The retrospective method and multivariate analysis allows use of large samples, which should enhance the statistical power of the results. However, key categories are not operationalised clearly in the report. For example, the category 'Asian' is not defined, and no examples of 'Asian' languages are given, so the measures of ethnic and language matching are not verifiable.

Evaluation of interpretation

There are limits to what such a comparative study can achieve without attempting to access the contexts and communication processes of the different programmes. However, the discussion of encouraging but limited quantitative findings raises key research issues for further research and development. The findings suggest that mainstream mental health services improve their effectiveness by developing a more communicatively and culturally sensitive service. The characteristics that differentiate the sensitivity of programmes have to be identified in relation to specific transcultural communication needs that may differ by region, ethnic and linguistic community, and health area.

Note

[1] Direct quotes are used to indicate researchers' choice of ethnic categories in the intervention studies, when the handling of ethnic categories appears potentially troublesome for the validity of the study. Related issues were discussed in the introduction.

FOUR

Intervention studies: advocates and linkworkers

Bilingual services: advocates – themes

One aspect of developing ethnically sensitive services is the provision of bilingual professional support where appropriate. The four types of bilingual professional are: the bilingual clinician; the interpreter; the linkworker; and the advocate. The next study specifically aims to investigate the possible advantages of using health advocates for enhancing communication. The work of advocates is distinguished from that of other bilingual professionals in terms of definitions of roles, goals and accountability. A central issue concerns their affiliations to minority ethnic communities, and their claims to a degree of autonomy from health professionals.

Study 5

'Improving obstetric outcomes in ethnic minorities: an evaluation of health advocacy in Hackney' (Parsons and Day, 1992)

Subject

The study tested whether a health advocacy service would improve obstetric outcomes in women whose first language was not English, in Hackney, London.

Aims

The study aimed to evaluate a health advocacy project that was established both to provide an interpreting service and to influence hospital policy and practice. Specifically, the intervention tested the influence of health advocacy on obstetric outcomes in "non-English-speaking women".

Rationale

Ethnic differences have been demonstrated in obstetric outcomes such as birthweight and perinatal mortality. Linguistic and cultural barriers add to the risks for "non-English-speaking women" in maternity units. Evaluation of the Asian Mother and Baby Campaign highlighted the need for workers to receive bilingual support from services independent from health professionals. The Community Health Council in Hackney, London, responded by setting up the Multi-Ethnic Women's Health Project to meet the needs of non-English-speaking women. Health advocates would mediate between patients and professionals to make sure patients were offered an informed choice of health care, and to negotiate clinical or cultural issues, as well as to interpret. They were encouraged to view themselves as being "autonomous" "advocates for their people". Their responsibilities included booking new patients, following each woman through her pregnancy, and attending every ante-natal visit. The project had an impact on hospital policy and practice, for example concerning issues of racism and gender. Anecdotal evidence also suggested effects of improved communication on clinical outcomes, but there has been a need for firm evidence.

Methodology

The study was commissioned by the Multi-Ethnic Women's Health Project (MEWHP), and the design developed through community consultations. A retrospective comparison study design used geographical and historical controls. A thousand women with Asian and Turkish surnames delivering at the Mother's Hospital between 1984 and 1986 were identified. Using case notes, the study group was identified on the basis of spoken language and use of advocates. One control group consisted of non-English-speaking women delivering at the Mother's Hospital in 1979, *before* the advocacy programme. Two control groups were taken from another Hackney hospital, Whipps' Cross, where local authority interpreters were used instead of advocates, one from 1979 and one from 1986. Outcome measures were devised, and the data collection form based partly on obstetric records. Results were analysed for differences in outcomes between hospitals, and historically within the hospital.

Intervention details

A randomised controlled trial (RCT) was not considered ethical because health advocates also provided an essential interpreting service at the Mother's Hospital, and because of the likelihood of contamination since the advocacy project had influenced hospital policy and practice.

Participants, dates and setting

The retrospective study was carried out after 1986. Women with Asian and Turkish surnames who were recorded in the case notes as 'non-English-speaking' were included. The intervention group cases were taken from the records of the 923 women identified as having delivered at the Mother's Hospital after 1980 (95% being from 1985 and 1986). For the control groups, 993 women were found who had delivered at Whipps' Cross after 1980 (70% from 1985-86), 866 who had delivered at the Mother's Hospital before 1980, and 999 who had delivered at Whipps' Cross before 1980.

Outcome measures

The following measures were recorded:

- method of feeding at discharge and six-week postnatal check (breast, bottle, or mixed);
- number of antenatal appointments not attended;
- length of antenatal stay;
  proportion of women aged 37 or over accepting amniocentesis;
- induction rates and Caesarean section rates;
- differences in birthweights recorded 'for interest'.

Results

Measures of frequency of use: overall, the study showed statistically significant differences between intervention and control groups in three sets of outcomes: antenatal length of stay, onset of labour, and mode of delivery.

There was an intervention effect on the length of antenatal stay. At the Mother's Hospital the average length was reduced from 8.6 days to 5.7 days, whereas at Whipps' Cross the length stayed the same during both time periods (5.7 days).

There was an intervention effect on the induction rate and on the elective Caesarean section rate. The Caesarean rate rose at Whipps' Cross from 2.9% to 5.9%, and fell slightly at the Mother's Hospital from 3.4% to 2.35%. Overall, the proportion of induced labours at Whipps' Cross rose from 14.4% to 16.1%, but remained the same (9%) at the Mother's Hospital.

There was only tentative evidence of an intervention effect on the proportion of antenatal admissions, and no evidence of an effect on earlier bookings, on non-attendance rate over time, on acceptance of amniocentesis, or on birthweight.

Interpretations

The authors note possible intervening influences other than the advocacy service such as technology and resource changes. However, the use of both geographical and historical controls provides some checks over this.

Flaws of retrospective comparative studies need to be considered. When selecting cases by names, it is possible that some poor English speakers who use advocates will be missed and some good English speakers who do not use advocates will be included. The use of advocates' case notes to record information is also a source of potential bias. An RCT is needed to provide further evidence that an advocacy scheme is a good buy.

Evaluation

The aims of the study are stated clearly and, given ethical concerns of researching advocates who performed an essential service, the method used seems to be the only choice. There is no evidence of bias, despite the risks in using historical and geographical controls.

Evaluation of interpretation

The conclusion that evidence has been found of significant effects of the advocacy service on obstetric outcomes is important, and strengthens the case for employing bilingual practitioners in this area. Yet the retrospective design and use of health records provides no insight into the intervening processes by which the use of advocates might influence outcomes. In particular, the report leaves some ambiguity about the roles which the advocates were sanctioned to play. While it is stated that the advocacy project was started with aims of providing an interpreting service and influencing hospital policy, the advocates' work is described rather differently in a separate section. Advocates are "autonomous", with loyalties to "their people" and "mediate" and "negotiate" between patients and professionals. According to Baker et al (1997) such autonomy distinguishes the advocates from linkworkers, who are employed by the health service and managed by health professionals. The absence of interview data illuminating this role ambiguity is a barrier to replicating the study or applying the intervention to a different target community setting. This omission is particularly problematic since the control groups were obtained from Whipps' Cross hospital which used "translators". It is important to clarify the different sets of work which advocates and translators might do, and their accountabilities, in order to identify conditions underpinning an effective advocacy service.

A strength of the advocacy project is that it was developed through community consultation processes, yet other cultural issues of communication remain unexplored. For example, the use of advocates from a community raises issues of confidentiality, and of working relationships with other professionals such as midwives, which are not dealt with here.

Bilingual services: linkworkers – themes

There is clearly considerable overlap between the functions performed by many advocates and those performed by linkworkers. Linkworkers in different settings may perform one or more roles within the health service, including advocacy roles, interpreting roles, and health educator roles.

Nevertheless a typical, if not universal, difference between advocates and linkworkers appears to be the greater autonomy of advocates in terms of accountability and line management, and the extent to which they are sanctioned to view their role in terms of service to their community rather than to the health profession. These differences provide a context for comparing the different studies reviewed in these sections. For example, the finding that a health advocacy service improves obstetric outcomes in women whose first language was not English (Parsons and Day, 1992) does not mean that a linkworker service would necessarily have the same effects. However, the absence of qualitative data analysis in impact studies impedes the clarification of roles and responsibilities that might account for success or failure. Of the three linkworker studies reviewed below, two (Mason, 1990, and Hoare et al, 1994) are impact studies using measures of knowledge and use of health services. Neither of these provides in-depth illumination about the roles played by linkworkers. A third study (Rocheron et al, 1989a) is not an impact study measuring health-related outcomes, but provides qualitative insights into the roles identified by linkworkers and other key participants.

Study 6

'The Asian Mother and Baby Campaign (The Leicester Experience)' (Mason, 1990)

Subject

As part of the Asian Mother and Baby Campaign in Leicestershire, the study evaluated the effects of using "Asian women" as linkworkers, in both hospital and community antenatal clinics, on "Asian" patients' health education knowledge, knowledge of available services, and use of health services.

Aims

The study aimed to assess the impact of a linkworker intervention on improvement of Asian mothers' use and understanding of health care during and after pregnancy. It also aimed to measure any resulting improvement in the health of babies, by measuring their birthweight and condition.

Rationale

Problems highlighted by previous research include inability of Asian families to use health services fully, due to the service providers' lack of knowledge of their needs, and due to lack of user knowledge of the services, and language barriers.

Methodology

Two linkworkers were placed in each of two city maternity units in the UK: the Leicester Royal Infirmary Hospital and the Leicester General Hospital maternity unit. Four linkworkers were placed in GP surgeries in the community which are described as "Asian practices". Pregnant women registering for antenatal care from 1 May 1985 to 30 April 1986 were included in the study. Women were interviewed on three occasions by questionnaire: in general practice when booking for antenatal care; on the maternity ward following delivery; and at the postnatal visit (six weeks after delivery). Health education questions were asked and demographic information and information about obstetric history collected. The design proposed to distinguish between a control group who did not see a linkworker, and three linkworker intervention groups.

Intervention details

The three post-hoc intervention groups were: those who saw both the community and hospital linkworker; those who saw a community linkworker only; and those who saw a hospital linkworker. Unfortunately, the report of results makes no distinction between the three groups.

Participants, dates and setting

The study was conducted in Leicester over two years from January 1985. Of 485 pregnant Asian women who were registered for the study, 457 (94.2%) remained in the survey sample; 407 (89.1%) completed the first questionnaire; 325 (71.1%) completed the second questionnaire; and 385 (84.2%) completed the final questionnaire. Of the total sample, 63% were Gujarati speakers and 17% were Punjabi speakers, with similar proportions in control and intervention groups. No details are given of the precise ethnicity, training levels or gender of the linkworkers.

Outcome measures

The number of linkworker contacts was measured in relation to the English language levels of the Asian women.

Antenatal care, delivery and health outcome measures were devised. The measures were: number of antenatal visits, admissions during pregnancy, gestation at delivery, birthweight, type of delivery, epidural rate and use of general anaesthetic.

Health education measures were devised for: knowledge of foods, knowledge of who to speak to for diet advice, understanding instructions, ease of explaining problems to a doctor, and preparations for feeding.

Knowledge and use of health service measures were devised for: dentistry routines, knowledge about postnatal visits, knowledge about the health visitor and contact routines.

Results

Number of linkworker contacts: approximately half the survey sample had limited or no understanding of English. In the hospitals, linkworkers were contacted at women's discretion. The result was that only 6.5% of women with good English had three or more contacts with linkworkers whereas 47.6% of women with limited English had three or more contacts.

Antenatal care, delivery and health outcome measures: there was no significant difference between the two groups in the time of attendance for antenatal care, nor in the other measures of antenatal care and delivery.

Knowledge of health education measures: baseline knowledge for all questions was better in those not seeing a linkworker than in those seeing a linkworker. Between the first and final questionnaires, where the linkworker group showed a greater improvement than the other group, this was mostly in those women with a good understanding of English.

Large differences between the groups were recorded for feeding knowledge. There was a 13% increase in breastfeeding knowledge in those who saw a linkworker compared with a 2% increase in the control group. There was also a 5% difference favouring the linkworker group in increase in bottlefeeding knowledge, but mostly among those with a good understanding of English.

The difference between the two groups in increase in understanding of written instructions was not significant.

Knowledge and use of health service: there was a big improvement (24%) between delivery and the third questionnaire in knowledge of "what a health visitor is" in the linkworker group, again mostly among those with a good understanding of English, compared with the control group (5%). But here the baseline knowledge of the linkworker group was less than 50%, compared with 70% for the control group. The linkworker group also showed a larger increase in knowledge of how to contact the health visitor (55% compared with 43% in the control group).

However, comparatively, linkworkers made no impact on dentistry use during pregnancy, nor, between delivery and six weeks after delivery, on knowledge of time and place for postnatal checkup.

Interpretations

The author states that overall the study indicates a small increase in the health education knowledge of women with linkworkers compared with the control group, and also an increase in their knowledge of available health services, yet there is no evidence that linkworkers increased the women's use of these. The linkworker group showed only slightly better delivery outcomes.

Most of the improvement in the linkworker group occurred among those with a good understanding of English. Similar improvements were seen among control group women with good English. Linkworkers did not seem to substantially increase Asian women's retained knowledge in areas of health services and education. More opportunities should therefore be provided for Asian women to learn English.

Evaluation

The aims of the impact study are clear, but a methodological issue is that since there was no randomisation, the linkworker groups started with a lower language level than the control group, which might have influenced their baseline knowledge levels. There would then be greater scope for an increase in knowledge in a group with lower initial knowledge.

The lack of specificity in the ethnic and language data about the linkworkers leaves uncertainty about the degree of language match provided. Nor is there much information about the work a linkworker would do. It is only stated that they were "facilitators" and "interpreters" while also performing an educative role. The initial design distinguished groups according to their contacts with community and hospital linkworkers but no further information is provided about this distinction, and the results are conflated into one linkworker group. Yet the impact of a linkworker intervention might vary by setting and by roles performed. Related to this, there is no account of how outcome measures were developed. Some measures appear decontextualised, lacking in cultural reference points, for example "Do you know which foods are good for you now?" The health outcome measures are not all in areas where a linkworker would be able to make any difference (for example congenital malformations). The report gives no evidence that the linkworkers were educating women specifically in the areas covered by the outcome measures.

Evaluation of interpretation

The claim that the linkworker intervention had a limited effect on health knowledge among the Asian women may be questioned on the grounds that the design is flawed. There is a want of clarity about the roles of linkworkers and the settings. The claim that the biggest gains occurred with women whose understanding of English was quite good does not seem to be consistently supported by the evidence. Specifically, the result for knowledge of breastfeeding indicates a stronger linkworker intervention effect than anywhere else, and most of this effect was in the women who had only a partial knowledge of English. Therefore the recommendation that there should be more attention paid to teaching Asian women English appears to be based on weak and conflicting evidence.

Comparisons across studies

By comparison with the advocacy study design (Parsons and Day, 1992) the linkworker study design lacks community involvement, and it lacks consideration of cultural aspects of health knowledge. Therefore the negative conclusions may be questioned since no consideration is given to exploring or meeting the conditions for effective linkworker transcultural communication practice. At the same time, the intervention also shares some of the limitations of the Parsons and Day study into advocacy practice (1992). The absence of qualitative components inhibits any 'culture-sensitive' understandings from emerging about how the goals and roles of the bilingual workers in their working relationships were perceived by the key participants.

Bilingual services: linkworkers

Study 7

'Can the uptake of breast screening by Asian women be increased? A randomized controlled trial of a linkworker intervention' (Hoare et al, 1994)

Subject

The randomised controlled trial examines the effects of a linkworker home visit intervention on breast screening by Asian women.

Aims

The study evaluates the effectiveness of linkworker home visits in increasing screening attendance, in areas where a high proportion of the population is Asian.

Rationale

Low uptake of screening is a problem in inner cities, while poor understanding of services is a barrier for Asian women. Communicating health information to women in their homes may promote better understanding and improve screening uptake, but there is a need for evidence.

Methodology

In Oldham in the UK, 527 Asian women, were selected for the study as they were aged between 50 and 64 and were due to be invited for breast screening during a six-week period during autumn 1991. Women with Asian names were selected from within seven general practices in the area with the highest proportion of Asian women patients. The study population was divided into Pakistani (n=324) and Bangladeshi (n=203), and randomised into intervention and control groups.

Two linkworkers were trained to follow up all women in the intervention a few weeks before screening invitations were sent out; second visit was made if necessary. Interviews were conducted in the relevant language using a semi-structured questionnaire to gain details of women's ages and addresses. An explanation of breast screening was given to inform the women and encourage attendance. The control groups received no visits. Attendance for screening was recorded.

Intervention details

In Oldham, the Screening Office uses a call–recall system where if a woman does not attend for screening following the first invitation a second appointment is sent. A health education leaflet translated into five main languages is included with the invitation to women with Asian names. The linkworker visits preceded the call–recall process by "a few weeks".

Participants, dates and setting

The two linkworkers were given "appropriate training". No information is given about their gender, ethnicity, age or linguistic background.

The Asian women in the study, aged between 50 and 64, were stratified into Pakistani and Bangladeshi groups.

Outcome measures

Measures of contact with the intervention group are given, as are outcome measures of subsequent attendance at the clinic for screening.

Results

Measures of communication patterns: in the intervention group, contact was made with 59% of the invited women, including 58% of Pakistani women and 62% of Bangladeshi women. Therefore two out of five in this group never received the intervention: Fourteen per cent were no longer resident at the given address and 11% were reported to be visiting Asia or only visiting this country from Asia.

Measures of health service use: no significant overall difference in rates of attendance was found between the intervention group (49%) and the control group (47%). No significant difference in rates of attendance between control and intervention groups was found for either Pakistani women or Bangladeshi women.

Attendance was generally lower for Bangladeshi women than Pakistani women and was affected by the length of time women had lived in Britain. Only 50% of women with less than five years' residency attended, whereas 73% of women with more than five years' residency did so.

Of 147 women interviewed in the intervention group only one woman could speak any English, only 17% could read in their ethnic language, and none could read English. Only 12% 'made any comment' when asked if they had heard of breast screening.

Interpretations

The authors state that lack of understanding of screening services is a possible barrier to attendance. However, the linkworker intervention of home visits was not a successful strategy. Contamination of the control group is possible, raising attendances overall, as the study sample belong to a close-knit community. Timing the intervention visit a few weeks before invitations were even issued may also have been a negative influence on the results.

Family support might be an important influence on attendance as 90% of women in the study said that they needed to be accompanied to screening. Also, there are difficulties in communicating the concept of screening women who feel well. The low uptake among Asian women might also be matched by low uptake among other women of similar demographic and socio-economic circumstances.

Evaluation

The RCT design is matched, but perhaps not sufficient, to the aim of investigating whether a linkworker home visit to "encourage and inform" would influence screening attendance. The possibility of contamination is noted, but the impact of the translated health education leaflet that was sent with the screening invitations is not assessed. Both might have been influences on the lack of significant difference between the control and intervention groups. The absence of ethnic information about the linkworkers, and the lack of data on the interactions between participants or perceptions of participants, makes it impossible to evaluate what possible reasons women have for non-attendance. Interview data might show whether there was contamination and whether the timing of the visit was less than optimal.

Evaluation of interpretation

The report mentions possible reasons for the lack of impact of the linkworker intervention but the study method provides no evidence-base for insights. There is a lack of information about the linkworkers' cultural attributes and roles, the perceptions of the women, and the social circumstances within which decisions are taken about attending screening appointments. Further research is called for which explores these factors.

Comparisons across studies

Neither of the impact studies involving linkworkers which have been reviewed above reached very encouraging conclusions (Mason, 1990; Hoare et al, 1994). However, neither study adequately questions the roles that linkworkers might play. In both cases it appears that they were expected to provide health information. There is little consideration of any cultural brokerage role, in bridging any divide between health service cultures and minority ethnic lay cultures. By contrast, a study reviewed below found that a combination of translated and culturally targeted materials (especially using video in the home) and personal contact by linkworkers appears effective in promoting cervical screening (McAvoy and Raza, 1991). But again, that study furnishes few insights into the processes by which women decide whether to go for screening. Issues such as family mediation of decision making and support for travel to the clinic need exploring.

The paucity of information concerning linkworkers' roles in these interventions is an obstacle for evidence-based service development, since linkworkers may be employed and managed by the health service. However, a fuller consideration of the issues surrounding linkworkers is provided in the study reviewed below (Rocheron et al, 1989a). Appendix 4, Table 1 highlights some key comparisons between these studies.

Study 8

'The evaluation of the Asian Mother and Baby campaign (full summary report)' (Rocheron et al, 1989a)

Subject

The study evaluates the role of linkworkers in the Asian Mother and Baby Campaign (AMBC). The campaign aimed to improve maternity services for Asians in 16 district health authorities between 1984 and 1987. The evaluation was carried out in three UK district health authorities: Wandsworth, Brent and Dewsbury.

Aims

The aims of the AMBC included encouraging early diagnosis of pregnancy and uptake of services; improving communication between mothers and health professionals; helping professionals gain the cooperation of Asian families; making Asian families more fully aware of the services and of reasons for using them; and ensuring that the services were accessible and acceptable.

The following aims of the evaluation directly or indirectly concern the use of linkworkers:

- to identify key factors in the linkworker scheme;
- to monitor any changes in the quality of health care for Asian mothers which are derived from the AMBC;
- to provide guidelines for future health education programmes for Asian mothers;
- to provide guidelines for training policies for health professionals delivering antenatal and postnatal care to Asian women.

Rationale

An aspect of the evaluation was the retrospective assessment of the assumptions underlying the campaign. The AMBC had two main foci, which provided a rationale for the roles which linkworkers were to perform: Asian mothers were to be informed of welfare rights and services, and health staff had to be educated about communication with Asian mothers.

Health professionals would define linkworkers' roles as health educators, and retain responsibility for them. Yet the linkworker also had to respond to patients' needs and rights. It was "stressed" by the campaign team that improving communication included raising staff awareness about Asian cultures and questioning racism. This last was not a publicly listed aim of the campaign, but during it, due to linkworkers' experiences, anti-racist training became a central concern. It was expected that pressure for change would come top–down from within the NHS, continuing after the project finished.

Methodology

In each of three evaluation districts, and in a fourth control district a survey of Asian and non-Asian adults was conducted before the AMBC started and six months later. Health professionals' views of the scheme were assessed through postal surveys and interviews with midwives, health visitors and linkworkers. Interviews were also conducted with Asian mothers.

Intervention details

Linkworkers were given one month's training, after which they were employed initially for a period of two years to work alongside health professionals.

Midwives' and health visitors' views of linkworkers were assessed by postal survey and group discussions. Completed questionnaires were returned by 129 health visitors and 106 midwives – response rates of 90% and 36%. Completed questionnaires were returned by 55 of 77 Asian linkworkers employed by the health authorities. A worklog provided quantitative data on linkworkers' patterns of work with each client in the three evaluation districts. Interviews were also conducted with linkworkers after two weeks of work and after one year. A small survey of mothers was also conducted. "Linkworker mothers" who had received help from a linkworker at least once during pregnancy were sampled in comparison to a retrospective sample of non-linkworker mothers.

Participants, dates and setting

The study was conducted over two years from September 1984 to March 1986. The three evaluation districts were the district health authorities of Wandsworth, Brent and Dewsbury. Home, clinic and hospital maternity services were included. The main participants were linkworkers, health visitors, midwives, and "Asian mothers".

Outcome measures

The study combines some quantitative survey analysis of user and professional service satisfaction and patterns of service use with more extensive qualitative analysis of observational and interview data on organisational practice, communication processes, and patterns of service use.

Results

Observation and interviews with managers: the impact of the evaluation district linkworker schemes was reduced by the absence of a prior local language needs analysis and of community consultations. Management were supportive, but prioritised the linkworkers' role in changing mothers' behaviour over influencing health professionals. Management had to work hard to sell the scheme to health professionals.

Postal survey of midwives' and health visitors' responses: overall satisfaction levels with linkworkers were high but varied considerably between districts. However, large proportions of professionals, for example 40% of Wandsworth midwives, were unsure of the aims of the AMBC and the roles of the linkworker. The differences in satisfaction ratings between districts and between different health professionals indicate the need for sensitivity to local influences on professional beliefs.

Attitudes to the linkworker campaign from group discussions among midwives and health visitors: midwives and health visitors generally agreed that linkworkers were valuable, while expressing reservations. Possible factors include resistance to linkworkers developing an independent role, which would affect the health visitors' or midwives' work. In fact, to do this, linkworkers would need more training,.

These health professionals seemed to lack sufficient training in skills of three-way interviewing.

Postal survey of 55 linkworkers in 14 districts: half the linkworkers had problems clarifying their role to health professionals. Around half "sometimes" came across "dislikable" attitudes of health professionals against Asians and around a third viewed these as "racist". The campaign team corroborated this with anecdotal observations of a depersonalised approach to care and overt racial prejudice.

Quantitative data in the logging system: there were major differences in patterns of contact between the three districts. Health visitors and midwives worked frequently with linkworkers but doctors rarely did.

Attitudes and experiences of linkworkers from interviews in evaluation districts: morale was affected by poor employment conditions, and there was a desire for further training. Tensions arose as all the linkworkers claimed that most of their time was occupied by interpreting, due to the health staff's demands, but they saw themselves as 'cultural ambassadors' as well as health educators and were trying to extend their role. They needed racism awareness training to deal with some staff attitudes. Linkworkers offered professionals linguistic help, and also served a cultural brokerage function. On behalf of patients they claimed to have interpreted, produced health education materials, and provided emotional and practical support.

Survey of attitudes and experiences of mothers: the "majority" of "linkworker mothers" felt that "linkworkers were there to provide ease and comfort to Asian mothers in an unfamiliar situation". About a half also saw linkworkers as "health educators". These roles differ from the interpreting roles envisaged by the health professionals. Linkworkers had provided a degree of continuity of care not enjoyed by mothers without linkworkers.

Outcomes

A number of claims are made, though without firm reported evidence. Health education leaflets and posters were produced. Parentcraft classes and family planning clinics were organised, and quality of information obtained by health visitors improved.

Interpretations

The authors state that overall the campaign focused on influencing individual behaviour, but there was conflict over linkworker roles. There is a need to specify a wider set of roles than 'interpreting' in job descriptions. Yet for clients a main benefit was personalisation of care and improved access to services. As the campaign developed, the aim of tackling racial stereotyping arose. Yet no sustained anti-racist policy emerged. The initial focus had been practical, and staff resistance and lack of community consultation played a part. The management structure excluded linkworkers.

Recommendations are made for different audiences.

Department of Health:
• Train linkworkers adequately, including advocacy skills. Produce guidelines concerning management and consultations with voluntary organisations.

Health authorities:
• Train staff in anti-racism awareness.
• Improve ethnic and linguistic monitoring of user needs and bilingual provision.
• Improve independent line management of linkworkers
• Coordinate interpreting and linkworker schemes.

• Ensure users have direct access to linkworkers.

NHS training authority:
• Improve linkworker salaries and career structure.

Evaluation

The descriptive aims of the evaluation are matched by the observation, survey and interview methods. However, the analysis of the views of different participants is based on very little hard reported evidence, and no evidence is shown of the quality of the intervention outcomes in terms of health education materials, or parentcraft classes.

Evaluation of interpretation

The study offers little evidence of linkworkers impacting on service use or health outcomes, but plenty of illumination into factors that might differentiate successful from unsuccessful interventions. The qualitative analysis of problems in the project provides a useful basis for recommendations about linkworkers' training and employment. The study shows that linkworkers may be thought of very differently by different health professionals and service users, and in different health contexts. The success of a linkworker intervention may depend on: community consultation; effective management in the context of sensitive issues; effective initial and ongoing negotiation of aims and roles; sensitivity to local histories and cultures; sensitivity to professional territorial concerns; adequate training; independent line management; and the attitudes of health professionals.

Comparisons across studies

The study provides insights missing from impact studies reviewed above (Mason, 1990; Hoare et al, 1994). The impact studies fail to consider the qualities of the linkworkers, roles they might perform, and the cultural sensitivities of participants, as influences on communication. The issues raised by this evaluation suggest the need for such qualitative work in preparing the ground for effective service development using linkworkers. Yet the current study also has methodological flaws. These include lack of rigour in separating evidence from evaluation, and contradictions in reporting (for example claiming that most health professionals approved of the linkworkers, while piling up anecdotal examples of resistance to their arrival, and mistrust of their cultural brokerage roles). Appendix 4, Table 1 highlights some key comparisons between these studies.

FIVE

Intervention studies: interpreters

Bilingual services: interpreters – themes

Several studies (for example, Baker et al, 1996; Hornberger et al, 1996; Baker et al, 1998) examine the impact of different configurations of interpreting services on a range of outcome measures. Hornberger et al, 1997, for example, measure communication process and health professional and user satisfaction outcomes of a remote interpreting service intervention, finding positive effects. However, little attention is paid to cultural issues in interpreting, nor to professional concerns of the interpreter. Baker et al, 1996, find positive effects of interpreter use on patient understanding of diagnosis and treatment compared with patient understanding when an interpreter was wanted but not available. A related study (Baker et al, 1998) evaluated effects of current interpreting practices, finding that untrained 'ad hoc' interpreters provide only a limited amount of patient interpersonal satisfaction. However, the definition of 'ad hoc' is itself vague and limited. Overall, these interventions use a range of outcome measures that include dimensions of information understanding, interpersonal satisfaction, and communicative adequacy. Yet the experimental designs, and strictly quantitative approach to data analysis, limit the insights of these studies into effects of interpreting services on communication across languages and cultures.

Study 9

'Eliminating Language Barriers for Non-English Speaking Patients' (Hornberger et al, 1996)

Subject

The study, conducted in California, US, compares a remote, simultaneous method of interpreting communications between clinicians and health service users with a more conventional, proximate and consecutive method.

Aims

The aim of the study was to assess in a randomised design the impact of two language interpretation services on various measures of communication quality and quantity. The new language service is called 'remote-simultaneous interpretation', which involves interpreters being linked from a remote site to headsets worn by clinician and patient. Interpreters are trained in skills of simultaneous interpretation. In the traditional service, interpreters work in the interview room and interpret consecutively. The intervention measured effects of the different methods on frequency of utterances, quality of interpretation, and levels of patient, interpreter and physician satisfaction with the two services.

Rationale

Potential advantages of a remote simultaneous service over other services include greater coverage of different languages, and better quality of interpretation. No well-controlled study exists comparing effects of different language services on quality or costs of care.

Methodology

A randomised control study compared remote-simultaneous interpretation (experimental) with proximate-consecutive interpretation (control). The site was a well-baby clinic. Subjects were 49 mothers who spoke only Spanish and were in hospital for delivery, four pediatricians and three interpreters who were employed in the hospital.

The first well-baby visit was randomly assigned to the control or experimental service. Use of control or experimental service was alternated at each subsequent visit at two weeks, two months, four months, and six months. Of the 49 tape-recorded mother–baby pairs, 22 were seen at least twice and 27 only once, 13 in the control group and 14 in the experimental group.

Control visits had an interpreter in the room performing proximate-consecutive (traditional) interpretation. Typically, one person spoke at a time. In the experimental intervention mother and physician wore headsets in the examination room. In a separate room 100 metres away, an interpreter had a headset and a control panel linking headsets. The interpreter could use a panel switch to hear both the mother's and physician's voices, or one voice only. The interpreter could also control what the mother and physician heard. The interpreter interpreted the physician's or the mother's utterances simultaneously. Physician and mother heard the voice of the interpreter and not the voices of each other.

Each encounter was audio tape-recorded to assess length of visit, quality of communication and accuracy of interpretation. Three bilingual Spanish speakers coded tapes 'blind' to the interpretation method, after 10 hours' training. On first hearing, they coded the amount and type of information exchanged between mother and physician. On second hearing, they focused on accuracy of interpretation by the interpreter; 35% of tapes were evaluated by at least two coders to ensure reliability.

Physician, interpreter and mother completed questionnaires at the end of the study to compare their preferences.

Intervention details

The three interpreters had experience of proximate-consecutive interpretation. They received 15 hours' of training in simultaneous interpretation. However, there is no evidence that they had previously been trained in proximate-consecutive interpretation.

Participants, dates and setting

The study took place at the Well–Baby Clinic of the Santa Clara Valley Medical Center of North California. The intervention period was six months, excluding training.

Mothers eligible for the study spoke only Spanish and had been in the hospital for delivery of a baby. No details are given of the four paediatricians.

The three interpreters were recruited from 20 staff who provided proximate–consecutive interpretation throughout the hospital. The interpreters are described as "foreign born" with at least six months of interpreting experience. There is a lack of detail about the interpreters' professional and ethnic background.

Outcome measures

Coders recorded number and type of utterances by professional and mother. Utterances were coded as 'questions', 'instructions', 'explanations', or 'requests for clarity'. Coders also recorded whether interpreters translated accurately or inaccurately. Inaccurate utterances were coded as 'additions' 'omissions' and 'substitutions'.

Questionnaires were used to ask all respondents which service they preferred. Physicians and mothers rated their satisfaction with using headsets, and physicians also rated the services on measures such as meeting patient needs, and assisting in making diagnosis. Interpreters rated the services in measures such as levels of understanding, and efficiency.

Results

- The remote–simultaneous service had 16% more utterances than the control service per visit. Yet the average length of the encounter was almost equal.
- The remote–simultaneous service had 10% more total physician utterances per visit and 28% more mother utterances per visit than the control service.
- Of particular note, physicians made 18% more explanations in experimental visits than control visits.

- Mothers made 22% more explanations per visit, and also asked significantly more questions and requests for clarity in experimental visits than control visits.
- The remote–simultaneous service had a 13% lower rate of inaccurately interpreted mother utterances than the control service.

Most of the difference was accounted for in terms of omissions of mothers' utterances in the control service.

Measures of attitude: all the physicians believed the remote–simultaneous service was preferable in all categories. They noted improved eye contact, although headsets sometimes interfered with their work. Interpreters reported that the remote–simultaneous service seemed to result in better understanding. However, they preferred to work with the proximate consecutive service. Of the 17 mothers who responded to the preference questions, all preferred the remote–simultaneous service. It was noted twice, however, that a crying child distracts from hearing through headsets.

Interpretations

The authors state that remote simultaneous interpretation resulted in more utterances by mother and physician, and in greater accuracy of interpretation, than proximate-consecutive interpretation. Physicians and mothers preferred it, but not interpreters.

The unpopularity of the remote service with interpreters is a concern. Locating interpreters in distant sites reduces their capacity to assess meanings in body language and to clarify a symptom that may have culture-specific meanings. But the remote service may help physicians to be more observant themselves.

Other options were discarded. For example, proximate-simultaneous interpretation would require headsets, while remote consecutive interpretation is expensive. Further studies investigate impacts of distance interpreting on costs and health-related quality of life.

Evaluation

The aims of assessing the impact of the remote interpreting service on measures of communication quality and quantity are matched by the use of a randomised control method. The quantitative measures confirm the expectation that simultaneous interpretation gives more time for mothers and clinicians to speak. However, the measure of accuracy of interpretation in terms of additions, omissions and substitutions, though useful, is limited. There is no measure of cultural and body language components involved in translation.

There may have been some interpreter selection bias. It is not clear that the interpreters had any training prior to their training in simultaneous interpretation. It is possible that they were therefore better trained to carry out the experimental service than the control service. It also not clear how their ethnicity, as "foreign-born" staff, or their gender, matched the mothers'. Any mismatch could influence evaluations more significantly in the control service than the intervention service.

Evaluation of interpretation

The results of the study support the positive conclusion that a remote simultaneous interpreting service allowed greater frequencies of utterances than a traditional service, reduced translation error, and was popular with clinicians and mothers in the specific clinical context. Nevertheless, there are some reasons for caution. There is a degree of context-dependence in the study. Distractions such as wired headsets and children playing could lead to greater problems of divided attention in other, less controlled, clinical contexts. The different sub-components of alternative interpreting service configurations are not explored with great rigour. For example, the reasons given for not testing 'proximate-simultaneous' interpretation – that it would require headsets – could also be reasons for rejecting remote interpreting services.

The study design excludes any in-depth qualitative investigation of communication roles. In particular the professional dissatisfaction of interpreters with the remote service is not sufficiently explored. Also, the lack of background information about the 'foreign-born' interpreters selected for the study suggests that insufficient conceptual attention had been paid to the interrelationship between language and culture in communication. The study only speculates, without firm evidence, that relegating the interpreter to the 'back room' will allow the clinician to assume roles of cultural brokerage and to develop rapport-building skills that would otherwise be assumed by the interpreter. Such speculation requires qualitative and highly context-sensitive evaluation.

There is growing interest in remote interpreting, which can be viewed as a practical and cost-effective alternative to proximate interpreting in some circumstances. An example is the use by practitioners of the Language Line telephone service in the UK when unexpected problems occur, such as the arrival of users from a relatively uncommon minority language group. However, remote services such as Language Line offer traditional, consecutive rather than simultaneous interpretation. Further research is needed to evaluate such existing services.

Study 10

'Use and effectiveness of interpreters in an emergency department' (Baker et al, 1996)

Subject

The study examines the impact of interpreter use in a public hospital emergency department on Spanish-speaking patients' understanding of their diagnosis and treatment.

Aims

The main aim is to assess how interpreter use affected the accuracy of patients' understanding of their diagnosis and treatment plans. The study also aimed to gauge patients' perceptions of their ability to speak English and their examiners' ability to speak Spanish, and to assess the relationship between patients' and clinicians' language abilities and use of interpreters.

Rationale

Much anecdotal evidence suggests that the reliance of many hospitals on untrained interpreters results in problems of inaccurate communication, misdiagnosis and poor compliance. Not to call an adequately trained interpreter when there is a need is discriminatory practice. No studies have looked at the relationship between clinicians' Spanish fluency and patterns of interpreter use.

Methodology

Spanish-speaking patients attending Harbor–UCLA Medical Center, USA, were enrolled for the study from November 1993 to April 1994. Patients presenting to the emergency department with non–urgent problems were eligible. Prior to examination, a face-to-face interview was used to obtain demographic information, self-reported health, and anticipated satisfaction with the visit.

One week after examination patients were interviewed by telephone, or face to face. Patients were asked to report their knowledge of diagnoses, treatment plans, and follow-up appointments. They were also asked to rate understandings on a five-point Likert scale. The same information was abstracted from the hospital medical records. Patients were also asked whether an interpreter was used, whether they thought an interpreter should have been used, and about their own ability to speak English and their examiners' ability to speak Spanish.

Patients' responses were used to create three post-hoc patient groups: group 1, 'interpreter not needed, not used'; group 2, 'interpreter used'; group 3, 'interpreter needed, not used'. Language concordance between patients and examiners was also divided into three categories: good, fair and poor. Patients' self-reported understanding of diagnosis and treatment was divided into two categories: good to excellent, and fair to poor. Regression analysis was used to determine the effects of patients' self-reported English proficiency and examiners' Spanish proficiency on patterns of demand and use of interpreters.

Intervention details

Interviews were conducted in patients' preferred language by a trained bilingual research assistant.

Participants, dates and setting

Harbor–UCLA Medical Center is a public hospital in Torrance, California. Spanish-speaking adult patients presenting to the emergency department on an initial visit were enrolled from November 1993 to April 1994. Physicians and nurses at this hospital request interpreters on the basis of their assessments of patients needs, rather than following patients' requests.

Outcome measures

Measures of patient knowledge: patients reported what diagnoses they were given, what medications were prescribed, what dosing instructions they were given, what reasons for taking medications they were given, and what follow-up appointments were recommended. They also rated on a five-point Likert scale how well they understood what was wrong with them, and the treatment plan. The same information was abstracted from the hospital medical records

Measures of organisational practice: frequency of interpreter use was compared with assessments of language ability and need of patients and professionals.

Results

Measures of patient knowledge: patterns of interpreter use substantially affected patients' perceived understanding of diagnosis and treatment:

- Best results were achieved where there was no need for an interpreter and no interpreter was used (group 1).
- But use of an interpreter (group 2) was associated with significantly better patient self-perceived understanding of discharge diagnosis and of treatment plans than when an interpreter was not used but was wanted (group 3).
- However, with the objective measures, no difference in understanding was observed between groups 2 and 3.

Measures of organisational practice: interpreters were used more often as relevant language abilities of professionals and patients declined. But no interpreter was used for 101 (46%) of 222 patients who thought an interpreter was necessary. Overall, when language concordance was rated as 'fair', 34% of patients said an interpreter was needed and not used. When language concordance was rated as 'poor', 30% said an interpreter was needed and not used.

On only 12% of the occasions when an interpreter was used was a professional interpreter called.

Overall, therefore, there were many occasions when an unmet need for interpreters was felt by patients. When interpreters were used the standard of interpreting was uncontrolled. Aspects of language support were significantly associated with patients' self-reported understandings of diagnoses and treatment plans.

Interpretations

The authors state that the frequency with which interpreters are not called despite patients' perceptions of need may have a number of causes. Health workers have the power to make decisions which patients may not agree with. Clinicians with limited language abilities may overestimate their skills or perhaps meet their own perceived information needs but fail to understand information or social meanings which patients regard as important. Clinicians may think they have understood an interaction while patients do not think the same.

Patients' perceptions of their understandings of diagnoses and treatment plans were affected by the absence of interpreters. Yet objective measures suggest no improvement in understanding with interpreters. It may be that the interpreters were not used at discharge, or that the quality of interpreting was poor.

Adequate language concordance between clinician and patient was associated with good understanding of diagnosis and treatment. Several measures are recommended to improve language concordance:

- increase the number of health care workers who speak minority languages fluently;
- train more interpreters;
- train hospital staff in communication skills when working with interpreters;
- establish specially resourced clinic sessions.

Among the limitations of the study, accuracy of self-reports may be doubted. There is a lack of information on the proficiency of interpreters. The study focused on patient understandings, not on the accuracy of diagnosis.

Evaluation

The bundling together of several aims makes any limitations of methodology more serious. The method relies mostly on patient retrospective self-reports, of understandings, of language abilities, and of preferences for language support. The method shows that limitations of patient understanding are associated with the extent to which their communication support needs have been met, but it does not illuminate how language support influences understandings. Among the unexamined influences on these processes must be the skills of professionals and interpreters, and the complexity of the information exchange 'task'.

Evaluation of interpretation

Despite several limitations of the study, the authors' interpretations point clearly to the impact of communication support services on patient understandings of diagnoses and treatment plans. Recommendations for service development appear to follow inevitably from the findings.

Comparisons across studies

Unlike the study reviewed previously (Hornberger et al, 1996), which focused on relations between patterns of interpreter service, the quantity and accuracy of interpretation, and patient and clinician satisfaction, this study examines relations between patterns of interpreter use and levels of understanding of diagnostic consultations. A companion study, reviewed next, uses the same sample and design to assess relations between patterns of interpreter use and levels of satisfaction with communication (Baker et al, 1998).

Study 11

'Interpreter use and satisfaction with interpersonal aspects of care for Spanish-speaking patients' (Baker et al, 1998)

Subject

The study draws on the same sample as Baker et al, 1996, which is reviewed above. It compares Spanish-speaking patients' satisfaction with interpersonal aspects of communication in interpreter-mediated examinations and examinations without interpreters at a public hospital emergency department.

Aims

The study aimed to evaluate the effects of current interpreting practices on Spanish-speaking patients' satisfaction with interpersonal aspects of the patient–provider relationship. To do this, differences of satisfaction were compared for: groups of patients who communicated without an interpreter by choice; groups who communicated with the help of an interpreter (typically an 'ad hoc' interpreter); and groups who communicated without an interpreter despite wishing to use one.

Rationale

Shortage of bilingual health professionals makes it necessary for health care workers to use an interpreter. Yet use of untrained interpreters leads to numerous errors and consequent misdiagnosis. Lack of an interpreter, or lack of a trained interpreter, may hinder clinicians from understanding cultural factors and impede the patient–provider relationship. No study so far has investigated this issue.

Methodology

Spanish-speaking patients attending Harbor–UCLA Medical Center were enrolled for the study from November 1993 to April 1994. The same sample, setting and method was used as for Study 10, except that instead of using interviews to identify patients' understandings of diagnoses and treatment plans, a questionnaire was used to obtain their satisfaction ratings for the practitioner who examined and treated them, and the nurses and clerks they encountered during the hospital visit.

Multiple linear regression was applied to assess the importance of interpreter use patterns and other patient characteristics on interpersonal satisfaction ratings for the examining practitioner.

Intervention details

See Study 10.

Participants, dates and setting

See Study 10.

Outcome measures

Five measures of interpersonal aspects of care were used. These were: friendliness; respectfulness; concern for the patient as a person; spending enough time; and making the patient feel comfortable. All these items were rated on a five-point scale from excellent to poor.

Results

Frequency of service use: on the basis of 457 completed follow-up patient interviews, 237 patients were categorised as group 1, 'interpreter not needed'; 120 were categorised as group 2, 'interpreter used'; and 100 were categorised as group 3, 'interpreter needed, not used'. Among group 2 patients only 12% saw the hospital interpreter. Otherwise, interpreters were nurses (28%), physicians (22%), other hospital employees (27%) or family members or friends (12%).

Measures of satisfaction:

* Patients who did not use an interpreter and who said an interpreter should not have been called (group 1) had the highest satisfaction with their examiners' interpersonal skills.
* In comparison with this group, patients using an interpreter (group 2) rated the provider as less friendly, less respectful, less concerned, and less likely to make them feel comfortable.
* Patients with no interpreter who wanted one (group 3) were less satisfied than group 1 patients on all items. Compared with group 2, they rated their provider as less friendly, less concerned, and less likely to make them feel comfortable. They were also less satisfied with the amount of time spent.

Interpretations

The authors state that having an 'ad hoc' interpreter was associated with less overall satisfaction with interpersonal aspects of care than not having one and not wanting one. Nevertheless, not having an interpreter when one was wanted was associated with the worst overall satisfaction ratings. In this study, 88% of the interpreters who were used were 'ad hoc' interpreters, so the relatively low satisfaction ratings are not generalisable to trained interpreters.

Untrained interpreters may have poor skills in five areas: explaining the role of the interpreter; transmitting information accurately and completely; managing the flow of communication; managing the dynamics of a three-way relationship; assisting with closure activities. Further research is needed to explore whether the use of trained interpreters reduces these problems. The gold standard for comparison should be communication with a language–concordant physician. Outcome measures should include patient satisfaction with interpersonal care as well as accuracy of diagnosis, and patients' knowledge of treatment plans.

Evaluation

The study design allows the researchers to evaluate the impact of using untrained 'ad hoc' interpreters on patient satisfaction. But the category 'ad hoc' is far too broad, and the method does not allow any associations to emerge between different categories of 'ad hoc' interpreter, such as 'family members' or 'nurses', and patient satisfaction.

Evaluation of interpretation

A limitation of relying solely on a retrospective survey for assessing the quality of communication is that the rating categories have to be comprehensible to the respondents. Since there is no observational data on the professional–patient interactions, this results in a loss of delicacy in analysing communication processes. Categories such as 'friendliness' and 'respectfulness' may be relevant but insufficient to assess communication skills. The report makes inferences about the possible nature of problems in communication with untrained interpreters, but these are drawn from secondary sources. A further issue concerns the so-called gold standard for comparison. The assumption that language concordance leads to skilled interpersonal communication in a physician, regardless of training, should be questioned.

Comparisons across studies

The three different interpreter studies reviewed above complement each other by focusing on different measures: of understanding of information, interpersonal communication, and accuracy and quantity of interpretation. The finding of this study (Baker et al, 1998), that using 'ad hoc' interpreters did not enhance patients' satisfaction with the quality of care, appears to be endorsed by the study of remote versus proximate interpreters (Hornberger et al, 1996). In that study, clinicians and mothers expressed greater satisfaction with a remote interpreting service than an in-room service. However, it appeared from the report that the interpreters had been specifically trained in remote interpreting and in-room interpreting. The studies appear to show that interpreting services make a difference, but that the use of inappropriately trained or untrained interpreters is unsatisfactory. They therefore appear to warrant further research on the effects of training on qualities of interpreting. Appendix 4, Table 2 highlights some key comparisons between these studies.

Study 12

'An investigation of the adequacy of psychiatric interviews conducted through an interpreter' (Farooq et al, 1997)

Subject

The study evaluates the information gained by a psychiatrist working through an interpreter in comparison to information gained by a fluent bilingual psychiatrist.

Aims

The assessment compares accuracy of interpretation and the degree of agreement between two raters (a bilingual psychiatrist and an English-speaking psychiatrist who used an interpreter) about family history data and symptomatic measures of a patient's mental state.

Rationale

Surveys of British Asians attending UK hospitals show dissatisfaction with existing interpreting provision. Psychiatry presents specific problems for understanding symptoms. The adequacy of the interpreting process involves more than verbatim translation, and shortcomings could lead to underestimation of emotional suffering.

Methodology

A sample of 20 patients aged 18 to 65 was obtained. Ten of those selected spoke Mirpuri or Punjabi, with very limited English. A 'present-state' psychiatric symptom and a family history checklist were used. An experienced, qualified interpreter was selected. A control group of ten English-speaking patients was interviewed jointly by two psychiatrists, and ratings compared. Non-English-speaking patients were interviewed separately, with no more than a 12-hour gap, by the bilingual psychiatrist and by the monolingual psychiatrist with the interpreter. Interviews were audiotaped and the questions used were the same in both sessions. Transcripts were used to compare the accuracy of the interpreter's interpretations, and also the ratings achieved across the two sessions with Asian patients and English-speaking patients.

Intervention details

The interpreter was told that the study aimed to compare symptoms elicited through different modes of interview – she was not told that accuracy of interpretation was also being assessed.

Participants, dates and setting

The clinical psychiatric interviews were conducted in the UK, but no date or location is given. The sample patients had no cognitive or speech impairments. The qualified interpreter had more than six years' experience.

Outcome measures

A list of 'mental state' items and 'family history' items was used to compare ratings quantitatively. Measures of interpreting content analysis were derived from the data and are reported under Results.

Results

Measures of elicited knowledge of patients: no significant differences were found between the two interviewers' ratings for any of the mental state or family history items.

Measures of communication processes: the inductively derived categories of common errors made by the interpreters comprised 'omission', 'substitution', 'condensation', 'similar phonetic sounds', 'conceptual errors' and 'exchanging closed and open questioning'.

Single examples are given of each of the categories, although there are no quantities.

Interpretations

The authors state that the study quantifies the relatively minor extent to which interpreting difficulties impact on elicitation of information. The experienced and professional interpreter contributed to the elicitation of information by modifying questions and answers to clarify them.

Among the possible causes of distortions of communication, the cultural values of a professional interpreter and patients may differ, despite the shared language. Clinicians may also speak too fast, use long sentences, address patients in the third person, use unduly technical language, and ask questions in an unduly indirect or impersonal way.

Several recommendations are made:

- clinicians should address patients directly to aid rapport and establish control;
- questions should be kept brief and jargon avoided;
- non-verbal communication should be valued;

- a pre-interview meeting with the interpreter is recommended;
- tape-recording interviews can be useful for performance appraisal.

Overall, interviews with a qualified, experienced interpreter are a reliable method of collecting information and facilitating reliable diagnosis. But there is a need for larger-scale comparative studies with trained and untrained interpreters.

Evaluation

The aim of assessing accuracy of diagnostic information gained by professionals is met by comparing ratings of mental state and family history items. However, the categories of interpreting error are arrived at inductively from the data and are not supported by any theoretical framework, nor by quantification, nor by extensive qualitative evidence. No evidence is given of the gender of the patients, nor of the language and ethnic background of the female interpreter. This absence of detail detracts from the transferability of the findings.

Evaluation of interpretation

The findings suggest that with appropriately qualified and skilled interpreters, relatively minor semantic distortions of interpreting need not undermine the diagnostic process. But the authors' interpretations are not all grounded in the empirical study. The data analysis does not focus on sequences of talk viewed as interaction between participants, but rather on decontextualised, discrete measures, for example 'omission' and 'substitution'. However, the report then discusses problems and skills of interaction and bases recommendations on that discussion. For example, evidence-free insights are offered concerning interpreters' modification of questions and clarification of answers, and clinicians speaking too fast.

Comparisons across studies

Whereas the studies of interpreting services reviewed previously illuminate some of the effects of failure to provide trained interpreters on patient understanding of diagnosis and patient satisfaction, this study illuminates the positive potential of using trained interpreters for facilitating accurate diagnosis. Unfortunately, in all these studies the reader is denied sufficient detail concerning cultural and language matching of professionals and patients to assess the transferability of findings. Also, none of the interpreting studies provides extensive extracts from transcripts of interactions. Where participants views are elicited this is through survey questionnaires rather than any probing interviews. Yet interpreting problems requires a more context-rich evidence base. There is a need for further research exploring the skills of effective interpreting, and for impact studies comparing different methods of interpreting, and comparing the effects of trained and untrained interpreters. Relevance of measures of effectiveness should not be determined only in relation to direct clinical concerns (for example compliance, diagnostic accuracy) but also more indirect attributes of 'consumer' satisfaction (for example interpersonal satisfaction, enablement, and understanding of health plans and service options). Determining the relevance of research to user concerns requires user involvement.

SIX

Intervention studies: training

Practitioner training – themes

A fairly disparate group of studies examines the impact of practitioner training on various outcome measures. Two studies explore the impact of training clinical staff on uptake of interpreting services (Blackford et al, 1997; Stolk et al, 1998). One study examines the impact of a communication training module on medical students' communication skills (Farnill et al, 1997). One study measures the impact of a receptionist training package on uptake of breast screening (Atri et al, 1997). Another study trained local residents to research perceptions of psychological distress among Pakistani and Bangladeshi people in order to improve services (Kai and Hedges, 1999). Finally one report evaluates the impact of an interpreter training programme using a range of measures including professional use of interpreting services (Farshi et al, 1999). The number, aims and methodologies of these interventions leave many concerns about communication processes unaddressed.

Study 13

'Breaking down language barriers in clinical practice' (Blackford et al, 1997)

Subject

The study evaluates strategies instigated by nurses at two hospital emergency units in Melbourne, Australia, to work more effectively with interpreters.

Aims

The aims of the 'action research' project were twofold. First, nurses identified practice issues in their care for people of non-English-speaking background in order to make recommendations for change. Second, the nurses implemented practice innovations and developed educational programmes in order to improve their communication. Through the action research process an emergent aim was to increase "appropriate usage of the interpreter service by nursing staff".

Rationale

The autonomy and decision making of people "categorised as non-English speaking background" is compromised through cultural and communication difficulties. Despite the needs of patients, current practice in Australia does not require nurses to use professional interpreters.

Methodology

The "critical participatory action research process" consisted of more than one research cycle. In each cycle, exploratory research is followed by interrelated phases of "planning, action, analysis and reflection". This is a non-comparative, qualitative and quantitative methodology. Responding to advertisements, 18 nurses volunteered for the first problem–identifying cycle, and 26 for the intervention cycle, only one of whom also took part in the first phase. Research strategies included questionnaires, interviews and audiotaped focus group meetings. These were used to inform action plans. These plans were implemented, and new action plans were built on analysis and reflection.

Intervention details

Through the action research process issues for training were identified with nurses. Professionals were the gatekeepers for families' interpreter use. Nurses assessed communication difficulties superficially on the basis of whether simple questions could be understood. Many nurses were unaware of interpreting services, or acquiesced with medical hierarchies in requesting interpreters for doctors but not for themselves. Nurses viewed interpreter provision as a function of family problems rather than also of professionals' needs. Resulting from these issues, "strategic action plans" were developed and tested. Problem-based education sessions in working with interpreters were developed by nurses and researchers for in-service education. Audio-visual materials and information packages were developed, and staff guidelines for assessing and responding to family language needs. Arrangements were made for ensuring advance notification of interpreter need, and posters were developed for display in clinical areas promoting interpreter services. Effects of the strategic actions were analysed.

Participants, dates and setting

A total of 43 nurses participated in two hospital emergency units at the Royal Children's Hospital in Melbourne Australia, 11 of whom were from an "ethnic background". The action research was carried out by the nurse participants with researchers.

Outcome measures

There are very few outcome measures beyond anecdote. The study measured increase in interpreter use by nurses (a measure of service use).

Result

As a result of the education programmes and posters the interpreter service reported an 85% increase in demand for its services.

Results reported without evidence: the increased demand aided the interpreter services to provide a case to change the service profile to include a more appropriate range of languages. Anecdotal evidence showed more accurate decisions and earlier and better treatments were being made. Through using interpreters more, nurses had better knowledge of patient needs and were able to make appropriate arrangements and discuss preferences. The study also claims that nurses' understandings of the impact of their own attitudes on communication changed.

Interpretations

The authors state that the most important change concerned nurses' attitudes in reflecting on their own practice. Through the action research process nurses reflected on their own 'ethnocentricity' as a factor in poor communication. They had used exotic models, positioned minority ethnic patients as 'other', and marginalised them by not using interpreters appropriately. They identified their own needs in order to change practice. For effective practice, nurses need to argue for policy and structural changes. One change would give families awareness of their rights to use interpreters. Nurses need skills in working with interpreters, and in improving their communication strategies. The action research process enabled nurses to become more aware, and worked as a vehicle for strategic change.

Evaluation

The study has clear aims and the action research design is clear in outline. The model is unusual in the studies found here in that it involves health professionals in research, though not lay participants, and pays attention to the process of research as a means of attaining qualitative insights. However, the methodology of data collection and analysis is reported in insufficient detail. Results are reported almost completely without evidence.

Evaluation of interpretation

The discussion of the impact of the reflective methodology on nurses' awareness appears plausible. Yet the report suffers from potential bias because the nurses' accounts of the process are not presented as evidence and not allowed to stand alone, separate from the researchers' assessments.

Despite serious flaws of poor reporting, two interesting 'findings' emerge. First, the action research cycle apparently has an impact on professional awareness which could be harnessed for training purposes. Second, through the process professionals can both identify and begin to address training needs, and needs for organisational changes.

Comparisons across studies

This study differs from others in that it identifies an iterative process that could be useful for communication training purposes. However, detailed issues for training about professional–patient communication processes are not addressed. With the partial exception of Farnill et al (1997), such insights into communication processes are not available in the interventions. Appendix 4, Table 3 highlights some key comparisons between these studies.

Training medical students

Study 14

'Videotaped interviewing of non-English speakers: training for medical students with volunteer clients' (Farnill et al, 1997)

Subject

The study reports on an intervention in which trainee medical students are taught skills for interviewing patients of "non-English-speaking backgrounds".

Aims

The overall study aim was to assess whether a training intervention was effective in teaching interviewing skills to pre-clinical medical students. Additional stated training aims were to provide supervised interviewing experience with speakers of English as an additional language, and to increase students' sensitivity to multicultural issues.

Rationale

There have been recommendations that professional training in cross-cultural communication should be strengthened in Australia. Lack of a common language and culture between health professionals and patients may interfere with quality of care. One response to this has been the establishment of training for professionals in working with trained interpreters. However, professionals also need training in communication skills to assess whether an interpreter is required, and for situations where no interpreter may be required or available.

Methodology

The project was viewed as an innovative teaching development, and is a non-comparative developmental study. Eight groups of trainees, consisting of seven or eight students with two instructors, met for 16 one-hour sessions, over a seven month period in 1994. Volunteers from 32 language backgrounds were used. At each session, after introductions, one student would interview a volunteer for 15 minutes, recorded on videotape and observed by the other students in the group. The volunteer and the student would then be asked to comment, and the rest of the session was used for feedback involving use of the video material, including a focus on critical incidents, and demonstration by instructors. Each individual student would practice interviewing twice, with a gap of five months.

Evaluations were made in three ways. Volunteers in the second interview round filled in a questionnaire to assess their experience. At the end of the project students rated their competencies at the beginning and end of the course. A psychologist rated the videotaped interviews 'blind'.

Intervention details

The second-year students had already acquired basic communication and interview skills through first-year course work, using video and members of the public. The intervention differed from the previous training in that the first language of the volunteers was not English. Students were observers and participants in 14 out of 16 one-hour sessions as well as interviewers in two of these sessions.

The students were only asked at the end of the project to evaluate their competencies before and after the course. It appears that the volunteers from the second session who filled in the anonymous questionnaires were different from those in the first sessions, so volunteer assessments could not contribute to evaluation of how students had progressed through the course. However, the psychologist's blind rating of the two separate interviews for each student could be compared with the students' self-assessments. The psychologist viewed each video three times, and the first ten videos were re-scored four weeks later. Inter-rater reliability was assessed by a second rater scoring 20 randomly selected tapes.

Participants, dates and setting

The intervention occurred over seven months in 1994 at the Faculty of Medicine, University of Sydney, with 60 second-year trainee medical students. Students' first languages were reported as English (60%), Chinese languages (22%), Vietnamese (6%), and other European and Asian languages (12%).

Community volunteers (36 male and 53 female) were recruited, with an age range from early 20s to late 60s. Volunteers reported 32 language backgrounds including "several European, Arabic, Indian, Chinese, and other Asian languages". Their language ability ranged from "highly articulate" to "very limited".

The course teachers, and the rater of the videotapes, were psychologists, experienced in teaching interviewing skills. The course teachers and psychologist also co-authored the report.

Outcome measures

Communication skills: three sets of rating items were used by the students, the volunteers, and the psychologist assessing the videos. The language of the rating forms differs, in that the volunteer items are expressed in less technical terms than the others. Although the areas of communication covered by the three different sets overlap, the categories do not all match.

Students' self-evaluation categories include:

- providing introductory orientation
- avoiding jargon and idiomatic expression
- using simple phrases and sentences
- adjusting speed of speech to needs of client
- skill in clarification of misunderstandings
- quality of open questions
- empathic responding to content and feeling.

The video rating categories include:

- commencing and terminating the interview – 'two items'
- simple vocabulary and sentence structure – 'two items'
- structured enquiry
- facilitation of emotional expression – 'five items'
- positivity of response and respect for the client – 'five items'.

The volunteer rating categories include:

- how well did you understand the student?
- how fast was the student's speech?
- did you ask all the questions you wanted to?
- how friendly was the student?
- how well did the student understand what you said?
- how well did the student understand important feelings?
- how well did the student show respect to you?

In common, the three sets touch on listening and speaking skills and on communication of feeling (interpersonal meaning) as well as understanding of ideas (information meaning). In the students' and video rating sets the management of openings is suggested, and the use of appropriate vocabulary and sentence construction. However, while the student items have no equivalent for 'facilitation of emotional expression', the video rating items have no equivalent for 'adjusting speed' and 'clarification of misunderstandings'.

Results

Volunteers reported positive experiences overall, and in all categories.

The lowest rating at the end of training was for "how well did the student understand important feelings?" The second lowest ratings were for "how well did you understand the student?" and "did you ask all the questions you wanted to?" There were associations between the volunteers' confidence in being able to explain an illness and specific predictors including their ability to understand the medical students and the students' ability to understand their feelings. The volunteers' emphasised the importance of being understood and of students not speaking too fast.

Students expressed "enthusiasm" and rated themselves as more competent at the end than at the start in all categories.

An overall positive effect of the programme on communication skills was reported by the *video raters.*

The total scores of 39 students increased, two showed no change, and 18 decreased. Significant improvements were found in skills of structured enquiry, positive response and respect, and commencing and terminating the interview. No improvement was found in facilitation of emotional expression, and simplicity of language.

Interpretations

The authors state that the programme exposes students to a range of life histories from different cultures, and to a wide range of English competencies. The exposure, it is claimed, offers some protection against stereotyping. The project supports previous findings that structured teaching of communication skills using videotape can be effective. Concurrent experience or maturation could have influenced the results. However, the programme follows from a basic communication skills course, so gains are likely to last and to be largely due to the course. Results suggest that more expert guidance is needed in modelling the use of simple language, and more effective training is needed in emotional perspective taking and responding to a range of feelings under various situational constraints. Overall, the project resulted in high-quality teaching and learning.

Evaluation

The multiple assessment method matches the aim of assessing the effectiveness of a training intervention. Despite the limitations of having only single volunteer assessments and student self-assessments, the 'blind' video rating procedure is fairly robust. There is no evidence of analytic bias, the detailing of the method allows replication, and it leads to suggestive findings.

However, there seems to be a mismatch between the methodology and the linguistic and cultural concerns underpinning the research. A research rationale is to evaluate an intervention promoting transcultural communication skills. Yet the study focuses on more technical aspects of communication skills, without linking them with cultural considerations. The 'rating scale' approach means there is little evidence of student or volunteer feelings about culture and communication, nor is there any sample of talk from the videotaped interviews. Consequently it is difficult to assess whether the training process led to any gains in student sensitivities to cultural issues.

The detailed working through of categories also appears unsystematic. The video rating categories are most important, since the video rating methodology is the most robust, yet here, unlike the student self-assessment, there are no categories for interactional speech skills (for example clarification of misunderstandings, adjusting speed). Also, there are omissions, for example of non-linguistic aspects of communication such as body language.

Evaluation of interpretation

The study suggests the potential value of interactive communication training using video and volunteer user involvement. But the interpretative focus on the importance of exposing students to life histories from different cultures as an inoculation against stereotyping is not derived from the findings on linguistic interaction. The conclusion that the course has been successful seems warranted by linguistic evidence only – there is no evidence of gains in cultural communicative competence. A problem appears to be that the methodology and categories were not grounded in a rationale linking cultural and linguistic aspects of communication. The concern that students failed to use appropriately simplified language and that they failed to understand and facilitate patients' emotional expression also needs further elucidation.

Comparisons across studies

This study is, strikingly, the only one in all the interventions under review that are concerned with enhancing communication with healthcare users who lack fluency in English, to use a reasonably wide range of categories of analysis of communication skills. The intervention is also virtually unique among the set in that it concerns training clinical professionals to communicate. Like the study of one-to-one health promotion communication using flashcards – reviewed below- (Hawthorne and Tomlinson, 1997), this intervention needs to be viewed as a sum of various elements, some of which are not considered in any detail in the report. A different methodology might produce insights into how the combination of video performance, repetition after five months, frequent observation, peer discussion of critical episodes, and tutor instruction are experienced by the participants. The lack of detailed attention to cultural and contextual conditions underlying the effectiveness of an intervention is also noted in the review of an intervention using culturally sensitive video to promote screening (Yancey et al, 1995). However, the training intervention reported here, despite its limitations, offers a valuable starting point for research into transcultural health communication training.

Training interpreters and implementing an interpreter service

Study 15

'Evaluation of the Leeds NHS Interpreting Project' (Farshi et al, 1999)

Subject

The report evaluates the progress of the Leeds NHS Interpreting Project, which aims to train interpreters and to establish an effective interpreting service in Leeds, UK.

Aims

The project aimed to establish over a three-year period a one-year diploma/certificate-level interpreter training course. Explicit objectives included: to hold training courses; to set out guidelines for professional interpreters; and to establish a highly qualified interpreting service. An evaluation was commissioned to evaluate progress of the project, evaluate interpreting service provision, and make recommendations.

Rationale

Patients are entitled to clear communication in their own language.

There has been dissatisfaction with the widespread use of inappropriate or unqualified interpreters.

Methodology

The project evaluation used a multi-method approach. An open-ended questionnaire was used to identify the views of members of the project management team (PMT). The Leeds NHS Interpretation Service (LNIS) claim form was used to assess service utilisation. Telephone interviews were conducted with 42 group practices across the five Primary Care Group areas of the city. Quantitative data analysis was used to identify the ethnic mix of populations, and the levels of use of interpreters, and 'content analysis' to identify reasons for low use. A questionnaire was distributed to health professionals in the community and mental health trust, and in two acute trusts, to identify professional use and views of the service. The process of interpreting was assessed using overt observation at one health centre. The experiences of qualified interpreters were assessed through a questionnaire followed by focus group discussions.

Intervention details

The evaluation provides many insights into current service provision, and views of participants on service provision and on training. However, basic information on the training course is not provided. No patient views are represented. The observation of the process of interpreting was limited to two ten-minute observations at one health centre.

Participants, dates and setting

The three-year Leeds NHS Interpreting Project was established in 1994. The evaluation was conducted between November 1998 and April 1999. Training was conducted at Huddersfield Technical College. The four participating organisations, represented on the project management team included two NHS hospitals trusts, a community and mental health trust, and Leeds Health Authority (LHA). The three years of the project resulted in a total of three trained cohorts, amounting to 44 newly qualified interpreters.

The evaluation included data collected from the project management team, interpreters, and professionals in the trusts, and from general practices.

Only three members of the project management team returned forms. A total of 1,136 interpreter claim forms were analysed. Mainly non-clinical representatives of 42 practices were interviewed by telephone. A total of 52 questionnaires were returned by acute and community and mental health trusts' staff. The distribution of responses included 22 midwives, 16 nursing staff, five psychiatric nurses, four consultants, three health visitors, and two ward managers. Questionnaires were completed and returned by 31 interpreters, and 24 interpreters attended focus group sessions.

Outcome measures

Qualitative and quantitative data were obtained from interviews with health professionals and interpreters, and claim forms. Details were recorded of service organisation and practice, frequency of interpreter use, and professional attitudes towards training and the service.

Results

Measures of service organisation: project management team responses viewed positive, long-term driving forces towards success as being counter-balanced by short-term constraints. The need for a highly qualified service and the presence of highly qualified interpreters was offset by insufficient administrative support; lack of a central coordinator; resource problems; lack of strategic support; problems with the training; and unequal distribution of interpreters between services. The weakness of administration affected the failure of the PMT to maintain contact with qualified interpreters. Members suggest a need for a coordinator and central administration, a central budget, and raising awareness of patient rights.

Measures of frequency of use of service: from the claim forms, it was found that total expenditure on LNIS increased from £3,677 in 1997 to £28,052 in 1998. However, overall, 80% of the total claims was spent on two out of the 17 interpreters who submitted claim forms to the researchers. The most popular languages for interpretation were Punjabi (43%) and Mirpuri (25%). These languages were offered by the two most-in-demand interpreters. A concern is that interpreters offering less widely spoken languages were almost never used.

With some improvements, monitoring of claims by language need and specialist area could be used to ensure more equal distribution of workload between interpreters.

Primary care, GP services: general practices had no formal systems of monitoring ethnicity, and did not use the interpreting services, using family members instead.

Measures of knowledge and attitude among health professionals, and extent of use of interpreting service: 81% of the health professional respondents from the trusts had access to lists of interpreters and 73% reported using them. However, 35% of respondents (particularly midwives) were required to obtain permission to use interpreters – an obvious deterrent. While 46% of respondents reported no problems with the use of the service, the main reported problems were the out of date or inaccurate list, lack of direct access to the service, and doubts about the process of communication with interpreters. It is recommended that staff need to be made more aware of the service and trained in the use of interpreters, while access to them needs to be improved.

Communication pattern /processes in primary care: two ten-minute observations provided very limited evidence. There may have been problems of insufficient eye contact between health professional and patient.

Attitudes and experiences of interpreters: the organisation of the service came in for criticism both in questionnaire responses and focus group discussion. Unequal distribution of work was a problem, as 35% of the interpreters had had no requests so far and might 'drift away'.

The lack of interpreter representation on the PMT, low pay, and delayed payments were problems. A service coordinator was needed.

The course itself came in for some criticism, but details of the course are not provided. Serious discrepancies abound between trainee expectations and the limited post-qualification opportunities for employment and demand for the service.

Interpreters sought regular work for all. A code of practice is needed, there should be regular meetings for interpreters, and the service should be better promoted among staff and the public.

Interpretations

A highlighted issue is the need for better coordination of an interpreting service which is used by different trusts in primary and secondary care. Issues of payment and employment are linked to weaknesses of organisation and support.

Evaluation

The effectiveness of the service is shown in terms of frequency of interpreter use and professional satisfaction. However, patient views are not canvassed. The aim of evaluating the course is only partially met as insufficient detail is supplied about it.

Evaluation of interpretation

The report contains evaluative components that focus on service organisation. It appears that the development of the interpreting service has suffered from limited consultation and management representation both in relation to interpreters and to minority ethnic communities. The evidence of problems in professional practice in primary care is also particularly clear.

To evaluate the impact of a developing service comprehensively would require detailed information about training, about the processes of communication, and access to user views. But the report indicates major issues requiring further research, in particular concerning interpreting in primary care, service organisation, and the attitudes of health professionals.

Comparisons across studies

Among the different training interventions reviewed in this report, this is the only one to focus on interpreter training and interpreting services. Unfortunately, as with other educational interventions (Blackford et al, 1997, Stolk et al, 1998), little evidence of training content or process is provided. The evaluation of the impact of the project on practice considers both resource utilisation and quality assurance issues, unlike other studies that exclude one or other dimension. However, the quality assurance dimension is not treated in depth.

Professional training and management policy intervention to encourage interpreter use

Study 16

'Lowering the language barrier in an acute psychiatric setting' (Stolk et al, 1998)

Subject

The study examines the effectiveness of training clinical psychiatric staff on Language Other Than English (LOTE) communications with patients in three psychiatric inpatient units in Melbourne, Australia.

Aims

The study aimed to discover whether a policy and training intervention would result in an increase in the number and length of communications with patients in languages other than English. The policy aspect involved senior staff endorsing the rights of patients with low English proficiency to use language services. The training aspect involved a "standard" training package for staff in the use of interpreters.

Rationale

Language barriers still hinder psychiatric service delivery to people who lack fluency in English. Previous research in Australia shows poor language matching of bilingual staff to clients, low use of professional interpreters when needed, and low levels of skills of many health professionals for working with interpreters. Ineffective communication raises the risks of misdiagnosis and ineffective treatment.

Methodology

A before and after study was used to measure whether LOTE contacts increased after training. A survey was used to assess staff professional experience, ethnic background, languages spoken, and professional ability in a lead language other than English. Patients' country of birth, preferred language, self- and staff-assessed English proficiency, and self-assessed need for interpreter were monitored. The outcome measures were quantity of interpreter bookings and booking duration. Communications were recorded in a four-week baseline period and a six-week post-intervention phase. Training sessions in working with interpreters were conducted in weeks five to six of the study. The sessions were repeated four times over 11 days with the result that 47 staff (59%) attended. Long-term effects of the intervention were also assessed over six months after the post-intervention phase.

Intervention details

The training sessions, a standard training package, lasted 90 minutes, and were led by the Victoria Interpreter and Translating Service. The training covered a range of issues including:

- the isolation experienced by 'patients with low English proficiency'
- booking of interpreters
- qualification standards of mental health interpreters
- guidance for using the two hour booking period
- issues surrounding the use of untrained interpreters
- interpreter roles
- staff skills
- confidentiality issues.

The policy intervention required unit managers to instruct staff to arrange three interpreter bookings in the first week when a patient with low English proficiency was admitted. The need for further bookings was to be assessed weekly. Posters displayed on the wards reminded staff when to use interpreters.

Participants, dates and setting

The settings were two inpatient units and a high dependency unit for acute psychiatric patients in Melbourne, Australia. Altogether, 80 clinical staff participated (including 10 medical staff, 58 nurses, seven allied health staff and five psychiatric service officers). Of the 80 staff, 48.8% (39) responded to the questionnaire assessing language skills; 28.2% of respondents were "non-English-speaking background-born" (NESB-born), 38.5% were "born of at least one NESB parent" and 43.6% were bilingual.

The study included all of 257 patients occupying beds during the 12-week study period between July to October 1995. Over half, 57.6%, were male; and 32.7% of all admissions were NESB-born. Of the 84 NESB patients, 49 (58.3%) preferred to speak a LOTE, self-assessments of English proficiency were available for 60 (71.4%) and staff assessments for 57 (67.9%). Of 60 patients, 26 (43.3%) rated themselves as having low English proficiency and 27 of 57 patients (47.4%) were rated by staff as having low proficiency. Of these 27, 24 were assigned an interpreter by staff, but three were not rated as needing an interpreter.

Of 11 languages that patients preferred to speak, four were not spoken by any staff.

Outcome measures

The number of LOTE communications (other than brief greetings), and also contact duration, were recorded. The contact form for each patient recorded whether contact was with a bilingual staff member or an interpreter, and language spoken.

Results

Measures of communication patterns/processes: the intervention resulted in a significant increase in frequency and length of interpreter bookings. Bilingual staff contacts showed no significant increase.

Almost half, 48.3%, of 'bed-days' of patients with low proficiency occurred post training, whereas 83.7% of interpreter contacts occurred post training. Since 48.3% would be a 'no-effect' result, the intervention resulted in a significant increase in frequency of interpreter contacts. Interpreter bookings increased from once every 53 'bed-days' preintervention to once every 10 'bed-days' post-intervention. There was no significant increase in bilingual clinical staff contacts post-intervention, however.

Follow-up data showed that interpreter bookings increased further to once every six 'bed-days' by six months.

Average duration of interpreter contacts showed a significant post-intervention increase from 51.2 minutes per booking to 85.1 minutes per booking. The duration of bilingual staff contacts showed no significant increase.

Interpretations

The authors report that the study demonstrates the effectiveness of the intervention in increasing interpreter-mediated interventions. The sustained increase in interpreter use at six months could be attributed to the implementation of quality assurance procedures to increase staff sensitivity to language needs; rating of language proficiencies on admission; the expectation that three interpreter bookings per week should be introduced for "low proficiency patients"; effects of posters; and management commitment to "culturally sensitive practice".

The fact that 41% of staff did not attend the training intervention causes concern. One year after the intervention some staff still stated that they were discouraged from using interpreters for budgetary reasons. Staff may need regular training rather than a single voluntary session. Bilingual staff still made the vast majority of LOTE contacts overall (75%) compared to interpreters. The data supports arguments for employing more bilingual staff.

Since the study was conducted in a naturalistic setting and with standardised training it should be generalisable, given commitment from unit managers.

Evaluation

The before- and after- intervention design matches the study, and the methods of data management also seem robust. A problem is the low attendance for training. Therefore, the significantly increased frequency of interpreter bookings may actually underestimate the potential impact of such training.

A difficulty is that the intervention apparently did not focus on bilingual staff, which may account for the lack of a significant increase in bilingual staff contacts. The primary focus of the training sessions was 'working with an interpreter' and the sessions were conducted by an interpreting service. Therefore, it appears that the intervention was well matched to the specific aim of enhancing communication with interpreters, but less well matched to the more broad aim of increasing the number and frequency of LOTE communications with patients.

A further limitation of the methodology is that it provides no insights into the impact of the course on the quality and process of interactions. Such insights appear required by the stated research rationale that many health professionals lack the skills to work effectively with interpreters and the concomitant risks of misdiagnosis. Indeed, given that course components included 'patient isolation', 'role of interpreter in patient–clinician communication', 'staff skills' and 'confidentiality issues', a qualitative approach seems fully warranted. There are, for example, no interviews, and nor is there any transcript data from communications involving interpreters.

Evaluation of interpretation

The authors speculate that continued success in enhancing interpreter use may be due to a combination of factors including the training package, the posters, management commitment, and monitoring of English proficiency. But the methodology furnishes no insights into the relative significance of any of these factors.

The study shows the importance of bilingual professionals, and room for further improvements in matching staffing to language need. However, the study does not illuminate the attitudes of the 17 bilingual staff nor of the other 63 staff to the intervention. Further research might investigate the most appropriate ways to promote inclusiveness in staff training.

Comparisons across studies

Comparison of this intervention with two others concerned with staff training in working with interpreters (Farnill et al, 1997, Blackford et al, 1997) shows the relative advantages and disadvantages of different approaches. In the intervention reviewed here the outcome measures supply evidence that the training package, combined with policy measures, leads to greater utilisation of interpreting resources by staff. This kind of evidence is useful for presenting a case to fund-holders and management for resourcing regular staff training in communication skills. The limitation is that no insights emerge concerning the effectiveness of the package and its component processes in enhancing the quality of communication.

By contrast, the Farnill study of a medical trainee programme using videotapes, does demonstrate gains in measures of trainee communication skills, though it is limited in its approach to the issue of culture, and unable to test long-term effects of training on practice. Some such approach is valuable since effective communication is a matter not only of resource provision but of quality assurance. The Blackford study aims to provide insights into the understandings of key actors, which are central factors in the effectiveness of any communication intervention, but unfortunately the report lacks evidence. From the comparison of the three studies, there is a need for communication training interventions that combine concern with increased resource utilisation and concern with quality assurance. At the same time there is a need to strengthen the credibility of research evidence by taking into account the cultural resources that different key participants use in managing and interpreting communicative events. Appendix 4, Table 3 highlights some key comparisons between these studies.

Training receptionists

Study 17

'Improving uptake of breast screening in multiethnic populations: a randomised controlled trial using practice reception staff to contact non-attenders' (Atri et al, 1997)

Subject

The study investigated the impact of a training programme for general practice receptionist staff on patient uptake of breast screening.

Aims

The study aimed to determine whether a two-hour receptionist training programme would improve breast screening uptake among women who had previously failed to attend, and whether different ethnic groups would benefit equally.

Rationale

Factors in inequitable uptake of breast screening may include social status and ethnic minority status. Studies have shown that general practitioners have not consistently followed up non-attenders. Screening rates appear better in practices with strategies to increase uptake, but there is a need for evidence of what strategies might work.

Methodology

Participating general practices in Newham, London, were randomised by practice, with fifteen practices in the control and the intervention groups. Practices were matched on practice size, previous uptake of breast screening, percentage of women aged 50-64 in minority ethnic groups in wards within a radius of 0.5 km from the practice, and the screening invitation batch. Screening appointment letters were sent batch by batch over eight months. A second letter was sent to non-attenders four weeks after the initial appointment. Non-attenders were noted, and ethnic group membership was recorded. A receptionist from each intervention practice was provided with a single, standardised two-hour group training session. The intervention receptionists were asked to contact all women on the practice list of non-attenders, and to record contacts made. Reports on attendance were collected at eight weeks after the last appointment in the batch, and periodically up to six months.

Intervention details

The receptionists' two-hour training programme "informed them" about the breast screening programme and "women's concerns". They were asked to contact non-attenders by telephone where possible or by sending a standard letter (in English with appropriate translation).

Participants, dates and setting

Twenty-six practices with 57 general practitioners participated; 12 practices formed the intervention group, and a receptionist from each practice attended training. Ethnic and language details of the receptionists are not supplied. However, in all but one intervention practice the receptionist could speak an "Indian language". Also, in 55% of control practices and in 68% of intervention practices the general practitioners spoke an "Indian language".

In the control group, 2,822 women were eligible for screening and 1,069 of these had failed to attend. In the intervention group 2,672 women were eligible and 995 had failed to attend. Therefore 2,064 women aged 50–64 were included in the study. Of these women 31% were reported as white, 17% as Indian, 10% as Pakistani, 14% as black, 6% as Bangladeshi, 1% as Chinese, 4% from other ethnic groups and in 16% of cases no ethnic group was reported.

Patients were invited for breast screening from January to August 1995. Attendance reports were collected over one year altogether.

Outcome measures

The study measured attendance for breast screening at general practices from a baseline of eight weeks after the last appointment in each "batch", up to six months.

Results

Of the 12 intervention practices three made no attempt to contact non-attenders. Contact was attempted for 646 (65%) of the 995 intervention women. Altogether, 314 were contacted by letter alone, 219 by telephone alone, and 113 by both letter and telephone. No contact was made with 349 women.

Measures of frequency of use of service: overall the intervention resulted in a 5% improvement in attendance for breast screening, while also showing better results for the Indian ethnic group than for any other. Of initial non-attenders:

- 40 of 1,069 (4%) in the control group subsequently attended;
- 90 of 995 (9%) in the intervention group subsequently attended.

Membership of the Indian ethnic group was also a significant factor in attendance:

- 8 of 149 (5%) Indian women in the control group subsequently attended;
- 40 of 206 (19%) Indian women in the intervention group subsequently attended.

This represents a 14% greater improvement in the Indian intervention group than in the Indian control group. In no other ethnic group was the gain greater than 8%. In the white control group, 14 of 372 were subsequent attenders (5%), and in the white intervention group 22 of 259 (8%) were subsequent attenders (a relative intervention gain of 3%).

Interpretations

The authors comment that the intervention had the most noticeable effect with Indian women. This might be attributed to the fact that most of the receptionists and general practitioners spoke fluently in "Indian languages". The improvements are viewed as modest but cost-effective. Training general practice staff to contact non-attenders could be used as a worthwhile part of multifaceted targeted programmes to increase screening uptake.

Evaluation

The study has clear aims with a broadly appropriate methodology, and the sample randomisation and matching procedures protect against bias. Therefore the finding that the receptionist training intervention led to an overall (modest) increase in attendance seems valid. There are, however, gaps in the report in two main areas. First, there is little detail of the training package. Second, there are gaps in the reporting of participants' ethnicity and language. Although the high proportion of receptionists speaking an "Indian language" is detailed, there are no details of what other languages were spoken by them. Also, although an overall numerical breakdown is given of the number of women contacted by letter alone (with translation if necessary), by telephone alone, and by both means, there is no breakdown by ethnic group. Due to both these omissions, the significance of verbal communication in a matched language cannot be assessed with any certainty. Consequently, only tentative conclusions can be reached about associations between language matching and screening uptake.

Evaluation of interpretation

The numerical association between the receptionists' command of "Indian languages" and the high uptake of screening by "Indian-speaking" women suggests the potential importance of language matching as well as training. However, the study only provides firm evidence that training leads to positive overall effects. While the authors suggest that such training could form part of a strategic approach to increasing screening uptake, a different study design would strengthen the evidence base for the approach. In particular, insights are needed into how different minority ethnic communities view health information and receive and interpret information about screening. On the basis of such information, an intervention might test the impact of different strategies involving receptionists. One such approach might compare the effectiveness of language-matched telephone approaches alone or in combination with written approaches or home visits.

Comparisons across studies

The study suggests the importance of training receptionists to communicate effectively with minority ethnic communities, to enhance screening. Several other studies have also suggested the impact on service uptake or on user attitudes of training health professionals to understand specific communication issues (Farnill et al, 1997; Stolk et al, 1998). But, as with most of the intervention studies, the report fails to offer detailed insights into how such training might work, either in its processes or its effects. Also, the intervention can be compared with two others (McAvoy and Raza, 1991; Stone et al, 1998), detailed later in this report, which show limited value in the use of either translated or untranslated written information in increasing screening behaviour when not supported by person-to-person contact. The receptionist training intervention fails to separate out the significance of person-to-person contact from that of written or combined-method contact. Yet the association between matching receptionists' and patients' language, and screening uptake among Indian-speaking patients, appears to suggest value in language-matched, spoken-medium contact in promoting screening uptake. However, doubts remain whether telephone contact would be equally effective with different minority ethnic groups with different language backgrounds.

Training and research

Study 18

'Minority ethnic community participation in needs assessment and service development in primary care: perceptions of Pakistani and Bangladeshi people about psychological distress' (Kai and Hedges, 1999)

Subject

The intervention trained local residents to research perceptions of psychological distress among Pakistani and Bangladeshi people in order to improve services.

Aims

The aim was to promote community participation in health needs assessment and service development by training residents to conduct qualitative research and to contribute to service commissioning.

Rationale

The importance of consulting with user communities about health needs is increasingly recognised, especially with the increasing role of primary care groups (PCGs) in commissioning services. Research has shown unmet needs in relation to psychological support and care of less severe mental health problems among Pakistani and Bangladeshi populations. Specifically there is a need to develop appropriate counselling services on the basis of better understandings of lay views of distress.

Methodology

The developmental, qualitative study focuses on how the process of training and supervising community project workers impacted on health needs assessment and service development. Local people from minority ethnic communities were recruited to become paid community project workers (CPWs). Of 17 applicants, 13 were recruited – seven of Bangladeshi origin, six of Pakistani origin; eight women and five men. The CPWs were trained for six hours a week over six months (over 140 hours) by a multi-disciplinary project team.

CPWs were supervised by the researchers in adopting an appropriate methodology. Semi-structured interviews were conducted in interviewees' homes using their preferred language. As a result of piloting, and CPWs' views as community members, audiotaping interviews was considered unacceptable to informants. Interview records and field notes were made by CPWs in English.

Recruitment relied on CPWs' networks, followed by purposive snowball sampling. Data analysis was conducted by the CPWs and a social science researcher. CPWs worked in pairs on data collection and pairs or groups on the analysis. Findings were then reviewed by community organisations.

CPWs reported to a steering group, which included a health authority manager, and two members of the primary care commissioning group. Subsequent feedback processes enabled project findings to influence service development.

Intervention details

The accredited training course involved small group work, practical assignments, role play, seminars, and a pilot study. Content included research methods and skills including community-led research, design, interviewing skills, and data analysis. Seminars were given on concepts of mental health, stress and counselling, and health service organisation. A module on methodology included issues surrounding research into stress in communities.

Participants, dates and setting

The study was conducted before 1998. The seven Bangladeshi recruits to train as CPWs were bilingual in Bengali and/or Sylheti and English. The six Pakistani recruits were bilingual in Urdu and/or Punjabi and English. The eight women and five men were aged between 22 and 39.

A total of 104 people from Pakistani and Bangladeshi communities all living within the "socio-economically disadvantaged" ward of Elswick, Newcastle, UK, were interviewed: 18 men speaking Urdu or Punjabi; 31 women speaking Urdu or Punjabi; 20 men speaking Bengali or Sylheti; and 35 women speaking Bengali or Sylheti.

Outcome measures

Measures of service development: the impact of community-linked research on local services is assessed.

Measures of attitude and belief: CPWs experience of training is reported but without evidence.

Measures of beliefs about distress and communication patterns: categories of causes of client distress and of coping strategies including communication are reported from client interviews.

Results

Service development: the community project workers completed training, gained an NVQ and carried out the research. The research resulted in subsequent initiatives from local services, principally recruitment of bilingual counsellors in non-general practice community settings, within six months. A programme was started to recruit bilingual welfare advisers. A programme of training in communication skills was started for local Asian people likely to encounter other peoples' distress. The model of non-directive counselling was adapted to be more culturally sensitive. A review of the NHS trust's mental health services for ethnic minorities was triggered. Local racism awareness training was prompted.

Communication patterns: study respondents located the sources of distress primarily in the external environment. In particular racism and socio-economic disadvantage were identified. A majority of respondents (81 out of 104) viewed talking to someone as therapeutic. However, a substantial number (56) preferred strategies that were socially orientated rather than solely focused on individual distress. They conceptualised 'counselling' as embracing practical help, for example welfare guidance and employment and housing advice.

A majority of respondents (75 out of 104) did not feel their general practitioner was an appropriate person to approach about personal or emotional distress, and most participants viewed the roles of primary care workers in terms of physical health and illness. Most respondents felt professionals offering help needed to give understanding and empathy, which shared language, age group and ethnic background facilitated. Gender was most important – only 11 respondents felt they would talk to someone of the opposite sex about distress, as this was culturally inappropriate.

Trainees' experiences: training and research was positively valued by the trainees. All the CPWs have progressed to continuing employment in a related area. The research revealed tensions between the steering group and CPWs, notably around taping conversations and obtaining biographical information from respondents. Trainees were attuned to community sensitivities whereas health professionals wanted detailed evidence.

Interpretations

The authors report that the work illustrates application of a community participation approach to needs assessment and service development. The approach could be applied to primary care groups. Training people from within a community to research that community has potential drawbacks. Among these are concerns about confidentiality, the possibility that insider perspectives might predominate excessively, and that an 'insider' might not notice certain aspects, for example of 'acculturation'.

Yet the approach has strengths. Use of CPW interviewers facilitates access and the development of culture-sensitive methodology. The process illuminates communication processes concerning illness, and has facilitated change at several levels. A culture-and context-sensitive research process might limit generalisability of findings but not transferability of the approach to other settings. The process leads to robust research, as is suggested by comparable findings of other studies.

Any compromise in rigour is balanced by insights into perceptions of need which provide a rationale for change.

Evaluation

The aim of promoting community participation in health needs assessment and service development is matched by the training and research process, which includes feeding back findings to community groups. Among the limitations that are noted, recruitment of interviewees from the researchers' networks contributed to age and gender imbalances. Information about acculturation was not sought due to confidentiality concerns of insider researchers. For similar reasons, lack of audiotaped evidence of interviews may have compromised accuracy.

Evaluation of interpretation

The evaluation primarily concerns the research process and implication of findings for service development, and not the quality of training. The evaluation convincingly illuminates some advantages and disadvantages of using community insiders for researching views of South Asian people on their communication needs when managing distress as a health concern. A major advantage is that the trust engendered by researchers appears to allow them to overcome potential communication barriers and gain valuable insights into user views of their needs and of the health service.

Comparisons across studies

The study provides more detail about the training programme than several other interventions reviewed in this report. The training course is also quite substantial – at least 144 hours over six months compared with, for example, a total of two hours of receptionist training in Atri et al (1997) and 90 minutes of staff training to work with interpreters in Stolk et al (1998). The lack of detailed course evaluation is a limitation shared by other training project evaluations (for example Farshi et al, 1999). The report is unusual, however, in attempting to describe how a training intervention ultimately results in culture-sensitive and language-sensitive service developments, aimed at improving communication.

Evidence of the effectiveness of training includes descriptions of a culture-sensitive research process, accounts of user needs elicited by the researchers from community members, and also details of service changes. But there is a lack of accounts from the trainees/researchers themselves, which limits the study, as it also limits the comparable study of 'action research processes' with nurse researchers/practitioners in Blackford et al (1997).

SEVEN

Intervention studies: health education programmes and resources

Health education programmes – themes

Two interventions (Brown et al, 1996; Elder et al, 1998) examine the impact of health education programmes on minority ethnic service users' physical health. The use of physical health outcome measures is unusual in the health communication interventions. There is a particular difficulty in examining possible relationships between a health education programme and physical health outcomes in addition to attitudinal, knowledge, or service use outcomes, due to the number of different possible intervening variables.

Study 19

'Initial results of "Language for Health": cardiovascular disease nutrition education for English-as-a-second-language students' (Elder et al, 1998)

Subject

The study evaluates a cardiovascular health education programme for adults enrolled in English as a second language (ESL) classes within adult basic education programmes.

Aims

The aim of the intervention was to assess the impact of the 'Language for Health' nutrition education programme, which was conducted in ESL classes in San Diego, California, on "low literate Latino and other-adult students'" nutrition-related knowledge, attitudes, behaviours, and physiological measures relating to cardiovascular health.

Rationale

Low literacy has a negative impact on health. The 'Latino' populations of the US contain a large proportion of recent arrivals many of whom are illiterate in English. Cardiovascular disease is the leading cause of death and disability for all groups in the US. Most current health education materials, predominantly using print rather than audio-visuals or verbal interaction, are geared towards educated and literate individuals. Most adults are also busy and need flexible learning systems. So adult basic education can provide a good opportunity for heart health education since students in ESL classes within adult basic education may be relatively motivated to improve language abilities and functional abilities at the same time.

Methodology

"Limited English proficient adults" were randomised into nutrition education and stress management ('placebo') classes. A randomised parallel group design was used in which an intervention group was given a nutrition and heart health education programme integrated into ESL classes while the control group received stress management education. Physiological measures and nutrition-related knowledge, attitude and behaviour measures were used at baseline, with three months' post-intervention and six months' follow-up. Participants were adults over 18, recruited from three community college sites during a one-week period in San Diego.

Participants were given "as many as" five three-hour classes involving culturally and linguistically targeted heart health education or else stress management education. Materials were learner-centred, culture sensitive and interactive. Seventeen ESL instructors were randomly assigned to deliver one of the two courses after a half-day of training.

A survey in Spanish or English was administered to collect demographic information, and attitudes, knowledge and self-reported behaviour. Data were analysed to measure change across time and between comparison groups.

Intervention details

The nutrition classes covered subjects such as understanding dietary fat and cholesterol; modifying cooking and eating habits; reading food labels; and understanding blood pressure. The stress management classes covered subjects such as defining and identifying stressors, and stress reduction techniques.

Participants, dates and setting

On three community college sites in San Diego, 408 ESL students volunteered and participated; 341 (86.7%) were "Latino", the rest "European" and "Asian". Almost half the sample was female, with an average age of 28.7, and 45% of the sample had lived in the US for less than three years.

Outcome measures

Measures of knowledge and attitudes to behaviour: the self-report surveys provided nutrition-related pyscho-social outcomes. These included scores for fat avoidance; nutrition knowledge; dietary self-efficacy; belief in change; intention to change; and (reflecting the placebo group's course) stress knowledge.

Measures of physiological change: total serum cholesterol and HDL cholesterol were measured. Systolic and diastolic blood pressure were measured. Waist and hip circumference were measured to compute hip–waist ratio. Weight was measured.

Results

Attrition: 69% of those enrolled completed the study. There was no differential attrition by control or intervention condition.

Intervention effects of health education: differential group change (evidence of intervention effects) was seen for five out of 13 dependent variables. *Measures of knowledge and attitudes to behaviour*:

- Fat avoidance scores increased only for the intervention group.
- The amount of change in nutrition knowledge was greater for the intervention group than the control group.
- There was greater increase in stress knowledge among the control group than the intervention group.

Measures of physiological change:

- The intervention group showed a greater increase in HDL cholesterol at the post-test, but by six months the two groups had converged.
- The intervention group showed a greater decrease in total: HDL cholesterol ratio at post-test, but again by six months the two groups had converged.
- However, six of the 13 dependent variables showed no differential group change.

Total cholesterol and blood pressure decreased similarly in both groups. Self-efficacy for diet change and intentions to change nutrition habits and weight showed a similar increase in both groups.

The pattern of results between groups for Latinos did not differ significantly from overall results.

Interpretations

The authors state that the intervention achieved only modest success, despite significant effects for fat avoidance and nutrition knowledge. Two possible reasons for this limited intervention effect are emphasised. First, the substantial 'secular' trend in the control/placebo group might be due to a Hawthorne effect. There might also be contamination between groups since many family members and friends were attending two classes concurrently and ESL policy left students free to drop in on other classes.

The study may not be generalisable to others of the same minority group who may be more 'acculturated', or too impoverished or stressed to attend such classes.

The study needs extending to include a measurement-only

comparison group. Using ESL classes solves some recruitment problems and offers a way of tailoring health education to participants' general needs.

Evaluation

There are methodological problems with this intervention. First, the attempt to randomise subjects to control and intervention groups within ongoing education programmes in the same college appears naive. The post-hoc discovery by the researchers that family members were represented in both groups indicates the inappropriateness of the methodology to an 'educational' research issue in which culturally mediated beliefs may influence outcomes. There is a strong risk of contamination as a source of bias invalidating the results.

Also, the stress management education programme may have been inappropriately used as an attention/placebo. Stress management could conceivably be a real factor in some outcomes, for example blood pressure.

Evaluation of interpretation

A concern is that the report concludes weakly that addition of a measurement-only comparison group should in future studies be used to overcome any secular trend in the comparison group. More fundamental questions need to be asked about the study. Although the report claims that the nutrition education programme was designed "especially for multicultural adults", no explication of cultural process or content is provided. The curriculum seems to have been developed without community consultation. The methods used are described as "learner centred, culturally sensitive and interactive" without any examination of what these terms mean, or whether culturally sensitive education methods are necessarily 'learner centred'. The list of topics covered includes no reference to ethnic or cultural dietary issues. The research methods preclude any insights into participant perspectives. The paucity of socio-cultural information about the sample group does nothing to allay concerns, expressed in the report, that the most disadvantaged populations may not attend ESL classes at all.

Health education programmes

Study 20

'Effectiveness of a bilingual heart health program for Greek-Australian women' (Brown et al, 1996)

Subject

The study evaluates the impact on various physiological health measures of a heart health education programme on a single community sample of Greek-Australian women.

Aims

The aim of the study was to assess whether a programme which introduced Greek-Australian women to appropriate physical activities, and encouraged them to reduce their intake of dietary fat, would reduce levels of obesity and improve cardiovascular health.

Rationale

Mortality from cardiovascular disease among migrants to Australia from Southern Europe is increasing. Regular exercise and healthy diet help to prevent premature mortality. Greek migrants to Australia and their Australian-born children show a strong tendency to linguistic and cultural maintenance. Therefore, it was important to develop the heart health programme with recruitment through Greek community groups to facilitate social support during the intervention.

Methodology

The intervention group of 26 women was recruited from a Greek Orthodox Church group to take part in the 24-week intervention. Physiological and self-assessment data were collected at pre-test and after 12 weeks of weekly group meetings at the church hall, each followed by a home-based exercise programme using a written booklet. Follow-up data were collected another 12 weeks later, during which time participants followed the home self-help programme only. A comparison group of 22 women was recruited through the Newcastle multicultural neighbourhood centre. They had little contact with the church group.

A bilingual self-report questionnaire was administered before the intervention to collect demographic information and assessments of physical activity levels and dietary habits. The intervention group was tested after 12 weeks and after 24 weeks in the following areas: anthropometric measures – total skinfolds, waist–hip ratios, arm circumference, changes in estimated percentage body fat, waist circumference, and hip circumference; resting blood pressure; exercise heart rate; self-reported dietary fat intake; and serum lipids.

The comparison group was tested twice at an interval of 12 weeks with no intervention.

Intervention details

The booklet for home use was written in English. It included a 12-week programme of aerobic exercise, and dietary and exercise information.

A fitness leader and a Greek-speaking health worker ran the group meetings during weekly two-hour sessions. Groups were conducted in a mixture of English and Greek. In the first part of the session that week's booklet material was discussed with verbal translations into Greek. Participants reported their shopping, cooking and exercise experiences, and discussed strategies. In the second part of the session practical exercises were done and assessment strategies were taught.

Participants, dates and setting

The study was conducted in Newcastle, Australia. The date is not specified.

The intervention group consisted of 26 women from a Greek Orthodox Church group. The comparison group consisted of 22 women from Newcastle neighbourhood multicultural neighbourhood centre. The only exclusion criteria were ethnicity and age (25-65). 'Good' English skills were possessed by 66% of the intervention group against 36% in the comparison group

The research team was all female. A bilingual Greek migrant health worker conducted questionnaire surveys and translated the booklet during the group meetings.

Outcome measures

A number of measures was used to assess physiological change after the 12-week programme and 12 weeks later. These included: anthropometric measures; resting systolic and diastolic blood pressure; exercise heart rates; self-reported dietary fat intake; and serum lipids.

Results

Of the 26 intervention group women, 25 attended subsequent tests, attending a mean of 9.2 of the 12 sessions; 21 of the 22 comparison group women attended subsequent tests.

Measures of physiological change
Anthropometric measures:

- Significant reductions of body mass index and total skinfolds were measured in the intervention group only, with no significant changes for the comparison group.
- A significant drop in percentage body fat was measured for the intervention group only.
- Significant weight reductions were measured for the intervention group, whereas the comparison group showed non-significant gains.
- However, waist measure and hip measure showed no significant effects.

Resting systolic and diastolic blood pressure: systolic blood pressure showed no significant intervention effects. The intervention group only showed a significant drop in diastolic blood pressure.

Exercise heart rates: a significant drop in heart rate was recorded at 12 weeks for the intervention group and maintained at follow-up. The comparison group showed a non-significant drop.

Self-reported dietary fat intake: self-reported dietary fat intake showed no significant intervention effects.

Serum lipids: there were no significant changes in serum lipids.

Interpretations

The authors state that the intervention had significant effects on body composition and aerobic fitness while the comparison group showed no change. The results show the potential of the programme to reduce cardiovascular disease risk factors through promoting modified diet and increased exercise. The success of the intervention is indicated by high adherence and low attrition rates and by sustained physical activity levels beyond the end of the formal programme. Two years after the end of the study, the Greek community still arranged exercise classes.

Factors in the success of the intervention may include the use of an existing community social group, running the course in a familiar setting, and the bilingual interactive format. The Greek women welcomed the chance to focus on their own interests and rejected the offer of having partners present. The bilingual format seemed acceptable. All the women spoke Greek by preference but they helped each other to read the English materials. The programme was appropriate in helping middle-aged and older women to overcome isolation, develop knowledge, and perhaps develop literacy skills. The participation of women with little spoken English can be encouraged by developing targeted programmes that address cultural and linguistic barriers to participation.

Evaluation

The aims of improving cardiovascular health and reducing obesity are well matched by the design and the range of outcome measures. A limitation concerns the absence of interview data to corroborate the plausible claim that having women–only groups meeting in a familiar setting, and using interactive methods, met the women's socio–cultural needs. A further concern is that the intervention group had better English skills than the comparison group. A group with lower English skills might benefit less from the use of English language home materials.

Evaluation of interpretation

Interestingly, the report emphasises that the evidence of lasting effects on the community is of equal or greater significance compared to short-term physiological measures. The study indicates how the impact of health education is mediated culturally and that understanding how that process occurs is a precondition of sustained or transferable success. Specifically, the report asks but does not answer what elements of the intervention could be taken up for mainstream service development.

Comparisons across studies

The ESL class study reviewed previously (Elder et al, 1998) suffers from difficulty of applying randomised experimental approaches to classroom curricula in a single educational setting, and the failure to consider in sufficient depth the implications of researching 'culture' in health communication.

By comparison, the Greek–Australian women's intervention (Brown et al, 1996) appears more carefully tailored to the targeted population group. While specific details may not transfer to other communities, the approach nevertheless indicates some sensitivity to the particular community's needs. The emphasis on collective mediation of learning and on sustained impact on a community also contrasts with the short-term and entirely individual outcome measures used in most studies. Appendix 4, Table 4 highlights some key comparisons between the two heart health education studies.

The study also goes some way to 'unpacking' a health education package, by providing a rationale for the different home and group meeting components. The importance of separating out the different processes and components of health education interventions has general application (see the review of Hawthorne and Tomlinson, 1997). Yet the unpacking would benefit from interview data. Such data for example might illuminate how women working together as well as individually influenced the outcomes.

Material resources and media in health education – themes

The next two studies examine the impact of visual materials and audiotaped materials on information transmission to minority ethnic users. The first study is specifically concerned with health education, with a focus on individualised teaching and learning (Hawthorne and Tomlinson, 1997), whereas the second study concerns the impact of tape-recorded assessment summaries on information recall (Ilett, 1995).

Study 21

'One-to-one teaching with pictures – Flashcard health education for British Asians with diabetes' (Hawthorne and Tomlinson, 1997)

Subject

The study evaluated the effectiveness of a targeted teaching programme using pictorial flashcards.

Aims

The study aimed to develop "culturally appropriate" pictorial flashcards for the education of "Manchester Pakistanis" with diabetes, and to evaluate their effectiveness when combined with a one-to-one individual teaching package, on patients' knowledge, self-caring skills and attitudes to diabetes.

Rationale

Previous studies have shown British Asian patients to have a poorer knowledge of diabetes than their white peers. Understanding of diabetes is a precondition of good glycaemic control. Pictures can improve understanding and recall.

Methodology

This was a randomised, controlled trial of one-to-one flashcard tuition followed by an outcome evaluation after six months. Pakistani patients were allocated to control or intervention groups at clinics. Sample size was 201 (intervention group 122, control group 89). Baseline questionnaires and blood tests were conducted before the intervention. At six months an interview questionnaire and blood tests were administered.

Intervention details

Ten colour photos of A3 size were piloted, and produced professionally with help from a dietician and a linkworker. The photos used Asian models, utensils and foods. Interviews were conducted by a linkworker fluent in Urdu, Punjabi and English, who translated the standardised questionnaire. The linkworker conducted the 'structured education package'.

Participants, dates and setting

The subjects were Pakistani patients with type 2 diabetes attending the Manchester Diabetes Centre and ten neighbouring general practices. They were enrolled between August 1992 and November 1993. Of the sample of 201 patients (94 male and 107 female), 192 returned for follow-up. Only five patients spoke English from preference, 70 (35%) had no formal education, and 66 (33%) had no understanding of English.

Outcome measures

Outcome measures were of knowledge, attitudes and behaviours, and glycaemic control (effects of behaviour on body health measures).

Knowledge measures included 'agreement on the importance of diet', 'knowing reasons for monitoring', and 'knowing diabetic complications'. Attitude and behaviour measures include 'hard to refuse food', 'can choose correct food at wedding', 'check glucose', and 'keep records'. Control measures were cholesterol levels and HbA1c measures.

Results

Measures of knowledge and attitudes: for the intervention group all knowledge outcomes improved. For example, at six months 78% of the study group could name one complication of diabetes compared with 18% at the start, and 16% of the control group. Some attitudinal outcomes improved. Most patients were positive about the "education they had received", approving the linkworker's "sensitive approach",

Measures of behaviour: self-caring behavioural outcomes improved. For example, glucose monitoring rose from 63% to 92% (no change for the control group). Glycaemic control improved, but there was no change in cholesterol. The control group remained essentially the same on most measures, except that knowledge of foot complications rose.

Interpretations

The authors state that low literacy levels did not prevent a pictorial education package in a one-to-one teaching programme from improving diabetes knowledge, increasing self-caring behaviour, and positively affecting attitudes to diabetes and the diabetes clinic. The intervention involved an integrated package of flashcards, one-to-one interviews and "reinforcements". Flashcards alone would be ineffective. The study describes an ideal situation in terms of time and language-matched resources (20 minutes of one-to-one education with a linkworker). Targeting is important as patients with high literacy might find the package inappropriate. Patients' attitudes, for example concerning disclosure of diabetic status when choosing food, were an important factor. But the support role of the linkworker could be important since the pattern of work might allow repeated contact. The study shows a linkworker from the community could be trained to provide health education in an effective way.

Evaluation

The study aims are not totally clear, as the report does not always distinguish the pictorial material from the "structured education package". Problems with replicating the study would be the lack of evidence of the content of the education package, lack of evidence of the process of education, and lack of evidence about the linkworker's "sensitive approach".

Evaluation of interpretation

The discussion introduces issues that appear to require further research in order to illuminate the conditions which made the intervention effective. For example, the linkworker is said to supply 'reinforcement'. Without the linkworker's 'sensitivity' the use of flashcards could be viewed as patronising, instead of empowering. The linkworker here is trained to provide a specific education component, but insights on 'sensitivity' and 'reinforcement' would be useful for training..

Comparisons across studies

The study leaves issues of content and process in education 'packages' unaddressed, as with the 'culture sensitive videos' study described in Yancey et al (1995), to be discussed later. Here, though, the preference of patients for one-to-one sessions is highlighted, which touches on issues of confidentiality also highlighted in, for example, McAvoy and Raza (1991). The importance of person-to-person contact, though not a finding of the study, emerges in the discussion. However, the linkworkers' roles remain under-explored (as in McAvoy and Raza, 1991, and Ilett, 1995). As with the other interventions that focus on materials, the methodology also precludes insights into participant views as an influence on their behaviours.

Material resources and media

Study 22

'Putting it on tape: audio taped assessment summaries for parents' (Ilett, 1995)

Subject

The study compares the effectiveness for parents of audiotaped, translated child development assessment summaries, with untranslated written summaries.

Aims

The intervention aimed to determine whether a tape recording of written child development assessment summaries was acceptable to parents and enhanced their retention of information about their child.

Rationale

Written reports of child development centre case discussions may not be intelligible to parents with poor literacy levels or who lack fluency in English.

Methodology

This was a comparative study. Parents of consecutive attenders at the child development centre at Birmingham Children's Hospital, UK, between 1990 and 1992 were randomly allocated to receive a tape recording of the written summary of their child's assessment findings in addition to the full written report and structured written summary that all parents usually receive. The control group received the written materials but did not receive tapes. Summaries on tape were in Punjabi, Urdu or English, while written reports and summaries were in English only.

Intervention details

The intervention was reported in terms of the impact of a communication medium (audio tape) on information recall and attitudes. However, a further variable was that the written summaries were in English. All parents were visited at home by an assessment team member after the assessment, with an interpreter "if necessary". Parents from the intervention group whose preferred language was English were allocated separately from those whose preferred language was Urdu or Punjabi. Translated tape recordings were made by a trained linkworker from a written translation of the assessment summary. Six weeks after the tapes had been delivered to the parents' homes, parents were interviewed there to assess their retention of information and their use of and views on the written and tape-recorded summary versions.

Participants, dates and setting

Parents of 113 children with Urdu, Punjabi or English language preferences were included, 83 families (74% of the sample) preferring English; five of these were of Asian ethnic origin. Thirty families (27%

of the sample) preferred Urdu or Punjabi. Of the 83 English-speaking families, 40 received a tape and 24 of these were interviewed. Of the 30 Urdu/Punjabi-speaking families, 11 received a tape and 10 of these were interviewed. The tapes were for home use within an inner Birmingham multi-ethnic population.

Outcome measures

The study measured parental recall of assessment team members, recall of recommendations made for their child, and preference for tape or written summaries. Reasons for preferences were also recorded.

Results

Measures of knowledge and attitude:

- Tapes led to no overall gains of recall. Use of a tape made no significant difference to recall of assessment team members' profession or name, nor to recall of diagnosis and recommendations.
- Preferred language of families made a significant difference to recall. English-speaking families had better recall of professionals' roles, better recall of diagnosis and better recall of recommendations than Urdu/Punjabi-speaking families.
- Of the intervention group who were interviewed, 43% of English-speaking parents preferred the tape, whereas 89% of Urdu/Punjabi parents preferred it.
- All Urdu/Punjabi parents who preferred the tape said this was because it was easier to understand.
- The results show that audio tapes make little difference to recall but that there is a language effect on recall in this specific context, with English-speaking families advantaged.

Interpretations

The authors ask whether the lack of improved recall might have been influenced by the lengthy six-week gap between sending the tapes and the interviews. The method is also impractically time-consuming.

Provision of a translated written report would have made it accessible to all the Urdu/Punjabi speaking families except one. The popularity of the tapes may be more to do with language choice than the medium. Yet video assessment summaries might provide an advantage.

Poor understanding of health roles and procedures may impede recall for Punjabi/Urdu parents. It may be that more effort is needed to explain professional roles, and processes and purposes of assessment.

Evaluation

The stated aims of the study involve testing a medium (taped summaries). However, it is difficult to assess what impact a medium might have on recall when another (written summaries) was available only in English. Also, information is not given about how users interact with the materials (for example repeated hearing or repeated reading). Such information could yield insights into conditions under which different media are used and preferred. Although translation is a likely factor in satisfaction ratings for taped summaries, the recommendation to focus on translated written material is unsupported.

Evaluation of interpretation

A number of issues are raised but not clarified in the report. The content and style of the summary report, and its clarity of purpose, could influence recall. Yet no sample is shown. This lack of focus on details of communication is a common issue in communication materials or media interventions. The report is also fuzzy in its account of person-to-person support. Professionals always make home visits after assessment, with interpreters available "if necessary", but this may be before or after the summary is delivered. So whether report summaries are then translated orally is uncertain. In any case, researchers and evaluators clearly need to separate out rigorously the medium from the language of health education materials.

Comparisons across studies

This intervention using an audio tape medium achieves inconclusive results. It is also not certain how far personal contacts had a bearing. However, the discussion of parental uncertainties about roles, purposes and procedures suggests that a combined media and personal contact approach (for example using a linkworker) might help understanding and therefore recall. In another study reviewed later in this section, combining personal visits and video health promotion facilitated screening uptake (McAvoy and Raza, 1991). To evaluate a culture-sensitive communication programme might require 'formative' insights into cultural processes by which users make sense of communications, as well as 'summative' outcome measures.

Health education materials and screening – themes

A group of interventions has in common the use of health information materials with the aim of increasing uptake of screening by minority ethnic users. Two of the studies show limited value in the use of either translated or untranslated written information in increasing screening behaviour when not supported by person-to-person contact (McAvoy and Raza, 1991; Stone et al, 1998). Two of the studies appear to show that video can be effective in promoting screening (McAvoy and Raza, 1991; Yancey et al, 1995). All three studies use experimental designs that are capable of establishing causal associations but which do not provide insights into the nature of any relationships between materials and behaviours.

Study 23

'Can health education increase uptake of cervical smear testing among Asian women?' (McAvoy and Raza, 1991)

Subject

This intervention compares different health education materials for their effects on cervical screening in Leicester, UK.

Aims

The study compares the effectiveness of different approaches to providing health education on the uptake of cervical smear tests among Asian women in Leicester who had never had a smear test. The study aimed to compare the effectiveness of using a video, a leaflet and a fact sheet. It also compared the effects of a researcher visiting to instruct the women about the video and leaflet materials (person-to-person contact) with the use of posted materials (the leaflets and fact sheets).

Rationale

Previous studies had indicated low uptake of screening among Asian women in Leicester as a factor in non-detection of cancer. Reasons given are said to be lack of knowledge or awareness, which would require health education.

Methodology

A one in 20 sample of women with Asian-sounding names aged 16–50 on 1 April 1985 was stratified by age, religion, and postcode area, and randomised into four groups. Two groups were visited personally and shown a video or leaflet and fact sheet. One group was mailed the leaflet and fact sheet and a fourth (control) group received no contact.

Intervention details

The intervention evaluated two main sets of variables. The first set was the three types of materials. The five-minute video had different soundtracks in English, Gujarati, Punjabi, Urdu, Hindi and Bengali. It consisted of a series of simple questions and answers about the cervical smear test combined with "appropriate" images and graphics. This was shown in homes with the researcher's portable video. The fact sheet contained virtually identical questions and answers to the video, and was also available in the same six languages. The leaflet described in strip cartoon format the early detection test for cervical cancer, again in the six languages.

The second variable to be evaluated was the difference between postal delivery of leaflet or fact sheet and personal visit for educational purposes. Although a research assistant was used for the personal visit, the visit would routinely require a health professional. Communication was made in the preferred language of each woman visited – only 34% being in English. An unanticipated 'problem' occurred in that, when informed that they were going to be shown a video, a quarter (42) of the women asked to be left to view it in their own time.

Participants, dates and setting

The subjects were a randomly selected one in 20 sample of women with Asian sounding names in Leicester aged 16-50 on 1 April 1985, and who were not recorded as ever having had a cervical smear test up 31 December 1986. The sample was drawn in February 1987.

Of the random sample of 737, 159 declined the intervention; 263 were shown the video; 219 were visited and shown the leaflet and fact sheet; 131 were posted the leaflet and fact sheet; and 124 were not contacted. The sample was drawn in February 1987. Subjects were visited in their homes between April and November 1987 and laboratory checks were made between January and March 1988.

The main languages spoken at home by the Asian women interviewed in the study were Gujarati (207), Punjabi (75), Urdu (36), Hindi (4), and Bengali (1). Overall, the study population largely comprised young married women of relatively disadvantaged socio-economic status by husband occupation. Of the 323 women interviewed, 223 had a video recorder in the house.

Outcome measures

The study recorded attendance for smear testing within four months of the intervention – a measure of service use. Respondents visited by the researcher were also asked by interview questionnaire for their views of the video or fact sheet.

Results

Measures of frequency of use/patterns of use of service:

- 5% of the control group attended the subsequent cervical smear test;
- 11% of the group receiving leaflets and fact sheets by post attended;
- 30% of the video group attended;
- 41% of those from the video group who said that they had actually viewed the video attended;
- 26% of the visited leaflet and fact sheet group subsequently attended;
- 37% of those from this group who said that they had actually read the information subsequently attended.

Of those who chose to view the video with the research assistant, 41% subsequently attended screening, compared with 64% of those who viewed the video alone or in their own time.

Measures of communication patterns /processes: in interview, 72% of the women who received personal visits with video made favourable comments, compared to 55% of those who received personal visits with leaflets.

The results therefore suggest that personal visits with videos were a relatively effective way of promoting screening for cervical cancer. However, visits with leaflets and fact-sheets were almost as effective. Postal methods were considerably less effective.

Interpretations

The authors state that the results would not necessarily transfer from Leicester to Bradford. The costs of personal visits would require a targeting strategy, perhaps focusing on women who had failed to respond to postal invitations (that is, on a call–recall system). Linkworkers could follow up non-responders. Home-viewed videos were effective, especially if the health professional left the women to view at their own discretion. So further efforts should be made to use video for screening promotion, perhaps also through women's groups and in video shops.

Evaluation

The study sample was carefully stratified, protecting against bias, and there is no evidence of contamination. The comparative design is interesting as two different sets of variables are involved (written materials and videos, personal visit and post) and not the quite common single-comparison control versus experimental design, which sometimes proves less illuminating.

Evaluation of interpretation

The study recommendation that videos be made available to women's groups and in video shops dovetails with concern about the conditions in which health promotion material is most readily accepted. The preference of 42 women to be left to study the video in their own time suggests the importance of user control over the conditions in which potentially intimate information is viewed or read.

Comparisons across studies

The recommendations that with a call–recall system non–attenders could be contacted by a linkworker with leaflets and fact sheets, or better still a video, are consistent with other interventions which support the use of video (Yancey et al, 1995), and which question the value of posted information without personal contact (Stone et al, 1998). The recommendation that linkworkers be used to provide 'personal instruction' and to offer to explain the materials also raises issues about the roles of linkworkers (as in Rocheron et al, 1989a). Here the linkworkers are viewed not as patient advocates, nor as interpreters, but as health education workers. The use of linkworkers without accompanying materials to promote screening was found to be ineffective in a subsequent study (Hoare et al, 1994). It is the combination of specific translated materials (especially video) and personal contact that appears most effective. But the study also touches on the desirable limits of such contact. However, the design affords no insights into the processes by which the women decide whether or not to go for screening. Also, as in most other interventions testing the effectiveness of materials, the paucity of reported detail about the materials is a hindrance to evaluation.

The results suggest the potential for exploring the roles of bilingual professionals in supporting women in this area, and that interventions need to draw on the views of the minority ethnic women on the health issues surrounding screening, and on educational materials.

Health education materials and screening

Study 24

'Increased cancer screening behaviour in women of colour by culturally sensitive video exposure' (Yancey et al, 1995)

Subject

The study tested whether culturally sensitive videos could be used in waiting rooms to increase cervical cancer screening behaviour among predominantly Latino women in New York and Los Angeles.

Aims

The study was a formal evaluation of English- and Spanish-language health education videos. Positioning the videos in community health clinic waiting rooms was believed to ensure that the target population – low income "women of color", with particular focus on Latino populations – could be reached. By placing the videos in two different intervention sites, the aim was to explore the value of the videotapes among different Latino populations.

Rationale

Previous studies had found that screening decreases cancer mortality, but that less formally educated and low-income Latino and African-American women of color screen less. Reasons are said to be lack of accurate knowledge of cancer risks and aetiology, and attitudinal barriers such as embarrassment. Fewer doctors' recommendations for screening occur with African-American and Latino patients. Factors include time, cultural assumptions, language barriers and social-structural barriers with lower income patients. As an alternative, the community health clinic waiting room provides an opportunity to influence patients directly at a 'teachable moment' of concern about health. No previous studies of the impact of health education videos in waiting rooms were targeted at minority ethnic communities. The video format can be used to emphasise relevant cultural dynamics. People from most backgrounds can understand it, and instruction can be combined with moving presentation.

Methodology

A quasi-experimental design was used. The one-week-on, one-week-off design was used at two sites, in New York and Los Angeles.

At William F. Ryan Community Health Center (Ryan) in New York, the intervention was conducted between May and July 1992, and at Venice Family Clinic (Los Angeles) between August and September. Videos were continuously displayed during two 'on' weeks in each site, to obtain a sample of 300–500. Two 'off' weeks served as controls at each site. Follow-up data were obtained from monthly laboratory summary reports showing the number of pap smears over three months at Ryan and over five months at Venice. Appointment rosters were used to identify whether more video-exposed women or more non-exposed women obtained smears.

Intervention details

The "culture-sensitive videos" were continuously shown on a 25-inch television screen. Women had the opportunity to see the videos while waiting to see the physician. However, there could be no way of knowing the viewing time for each patient nor whether patients actually watched. The videos ran continuously, "alternating Spanish and English" in each video, with a total running time of 50 minutes (35 minutes total on cervical cancer prevention and 15 on breast cancer prevention). The videos used interviews with members of the target population to explore feelings and beliefs about cancer and screening processes. Experts from the same ethnic backgrounds provided commentary and narration. Most patients wait between 30 minutes and an hour and so would have time to see most of a complete video.

Participants, dates and setting

The intervention samples were 335 at Venice and 533 at Ryan, the control samples 325 at Venice and 551 at Ryan.

At Venice 75.4% of the intervention groups were 'Latina' women, the majority of Mexican and Central American descent; 84.9% were "below the poverty line". At Ryan 55.7% of the intervention group were Latina women, mainly of Puerto Rican, Dominican or Caribbean descent. Poverty line figures were not available but 50.7% had no medical insurance.

Although language data is not provided, the Spanish language is claimed to be the most unifying characteristic of Latino Americans.

The waiting room settings presented potential problems. At Venice waiting room noise levels interfered with the sound, and the sound interfered with staff. At Ryan room shape prevented more than five or six people at any time having a good view.

Outcome measures

The study follow-up data were taken from monthly laboratory summary reports. These identified patients by name and patient ID number. Comparison with appointments records showed whether the women belonged to the video-exposed or control group.

Results

Measures of service use: the study showed that the proportion of women who received pap smears was approximately one third higher among those who were exposed to a video intervention than among the control group at each clinic.

The intervention effect was statistically significant at the 0.05 level (P=0.011 and P=0.016 at Venice and Ryan respectively).

Interpretations

The authors state that culturally sensitive videos significantly increase cervical cancer screening behaviour among the patients. But a number of limitations are noted. Age- and ethnicity-specific results are not available due to the 'ecological' design. Comparisons with other less culturally sensitive videos were not made, but the inefficacy of the latter is already documented. The study design does not illuminate the process by which referral increased. It is not clear who actually watched the videos, nor whether the videos had a significant impact on staff behaviour. It is also not clear what aspects of the video would have been effective. Language and culture sensitivity are the likely candidates. There may conceivably have been contamination as the control group may have heard of the video. However, the results could then have been more significant without contamination.

The intervention is low cost in resources and staff time, but it needs to be targeted carefully. Socio-economic status may be as important as ethnicity in the take-up of services. A strength of this study is its ecological validity.

Evaluation

The design has the advantage that two distinct settings are used and despite different intervening factors in each setting similar results were obtained. Although the control and intervention groups were not matched, similarities of ethnic backgrounds, income and age are clearly shown. The disadvantage of using a single outcome measure of service uptake is that insights into process are not obtained, and there is no evidence of how directly or indirectly the videos impacted on either patients or staff.

Evaluation of interpretation

The findings and recommendations concerning the potential value of a culturally sensitive video for health education and enhancing screening uptake are consistent with McAvoy and Raza (1991). However, the report provides limited detail of the culture-sensitive content, and affords little insight into cultural processes. For example, breast and cervical cancer might be viewed as delicate topics for public discussion, yet the video is shown in a public waiting room. The McAvoy and Raza study found that a considerable percentage of women preferred to view the video without an attendant professional. In this regard, cultural sensitivity concerns not just content but process. Mention is made of staff irritation at the noise levels and the repetitiveness of the video loop, and also of the noise of children next to the video equipment. So women accompanied by children are invited to watch culturally sensitive videos, yet there is no methodological attempt to explore the possible significance of these factors for the people concerned.

The encouraging results suggest further research investigating the transferability of videos as health education materials into different minority ethnic communities. But exploratory work is needed into specific minority ethnic user views of 'cultural sensitivity' in relation to their health needs and the processes of health education.

Health education materials and screening – themes

A finding of the McAvoy and Raza (1991) study was that translated materials sent by post are ineffective in promoting screening. A related study (Stone et al, 1998) looks at the potential impact of sending screening letters and information leaflets by post in translated and untranslated format.

Study 25

'Reasons for non-compliance with screening for infection with Helicobacter pylori, in a multi-ethnic community in Leicester, UK' (Stone et al, 1998)

Subject

The study compared the effects on attendance for screening for infection with *Helicobacter pylori* (H pylori) of sending screening invitations and information leaflets in English only, and sending screening invitations in English but with a brief translated covering note and translated information leaflets in Gujarati. The subjects were South Asian Gujarati speakers in Leicester. A non-Asian English-speaking control group was also sent the all-English version.

Aims

The study aims were twofold. The intervention was designed to assess the effectiveness on uptake of mailing information in an "Asian language" (Gujarati) and to identify reasons for non-acceptance of invitations in both "Asian" and "non-Asian" populations.

Rationale

The report states that the South Asian population is known to have a high prevalence of H pylori infection and peptic ulcer disease. An association between the two has been clinically confirmed. Screening is a possibility for the future, especially given the proven link between H pylori and gastric cancer, and the proposed association between H pylori and chronic heart disease. There may be a problem with "compliance" with screening in "ethnic minority communities".

Methodology

An experimental methodology was used with randomised groups for comparison. The sample frame was a list of patients aged 21-55 obtained from Leicester Health Authority. Asians and non-Asians were identified by name and a computer-generated random number list of 200 was produced from each group.

In stage one of the intervention both groups of 200 were invited to screen, using English language materials. Records were kept of non-attenders who had moved. The remaining non-attenders were identified and semi-structured interviews carried out to assess reasons for non-attendance. At a second stage a further matched group of Asians was selected from the same sample frame. Invitations were sent out with Gujarati supplementary material. Follow-up interviews were not conducted.

Intervention details

The invitation letters were sent through general practitioners. The letters stated that the screening programme was part of a research study, gave an appointment time, offered to rearrange that time if necessary, and mentioned that the test would involve giving blood. Also, the letter mentioned that those testing positive could request a prescription. Subjects were asked to mail a reply slip in a prepaid envelope to indicate whether they would come. A questionnaire was included which requested demographic and symptom details to be brought to the screening session. The report does not comment on the impact of stating that the programme is part of a research study, nor on the demands made of subjects by the letter.

The information leaflet was "specifically designed to be easily readable". The report does not show the leaflet nor provide further details.

At the first stage all information was in English. At the second stage the information leaflet was sent out in English and Gujarati versions, and the brief information slip in Gujarati explaining the contents of the letter.

Participants, dates and settings

Subjects were categorised as "Asians" and "non-Asians". The study was conducted within the catchment of a single general practice in Belgrave, Leicester, where Gujarati is the most commonly spoken Asian language. The only socio-demographic information provided is that the practice covers an area of terraced housing, while many of the subjects were employed in the knitwear trade. The research worker who conducted interviews was fluent in Gujarati and Hindi. Those randomly selected for each phase comprised 116 male and 84 female subjects aged 21-55.

Outcome measures

Reasons given for non-attendance were recorded from interviews. General practice records were used to identify non-attenders who had moved. Attendances at screening sessions were recorded from attendance records.

Results

Measures of service use:

- Attendances were low for all three groups.
- Using translated materials showed no improvement over non-translated materials.
- In the first phase 42 of 195 eligible non–Asians (22%) and 59 out of 200 eligible Asians (30%) attended for screening .
- In the second phase 51 out of 200 Asians (26%) attended for screening.
- 81 non–Asians and 65 Asians (34%) had moved address. Only 14 reply slips (eight non–Asian and three Asian) were returned giving reasons for non-attendance.

From the first phase, the main reasons given for non-attendance by those who had not moved were:

Asians (n = 70):
Too busy = 18
Family commitments = 10
Letter not read/not fully understood 9
Non–Asians (n = 61)
No recall of receiving letter = 12
Too busy = 10
On holiday/away from home = 10

All those Asians interviewed from the first stage had someone who could read in English for them; 13 of the 70 said they would take more notice if the letter was in an Asian language, but only five thought that this would affect their behaviour.

Overall, therefore, the results show few differences between ethnicities in the attendance levels, which were low. The translated materials made no difference.

Interpretations

The authors comment on the inadequacy of health records with an out-of-date list of addresses. They also conclude that language difficulties are not the most significant factor in the low uptake of screening. The report concludes that people were apparently not sufficiently motivated to read the letters. Personal visits might help with Asian and non-Asian groups, with a targeting of resources towards low attenders. More flexible appointment times might also help. Overall, there is a need for educational interventions to increase interest. This conclusion is in line with the rationale for the interventions using health education materials (McAvoy and Raza, 1991; Yancey et al, 1995).

Evaluation

The two sets of study aims are clear, and the ineffectiveness of the intervention is demonstrated. However, the study does not convincingly demonstrate reasons for non-compliance. The main reason for this is the non-ecological method. There is very little evidence allowed by the study design on contextual factors, such as how users understand their own wants in relation to their views of health and the health service.

Evaluation of interpretation

The discussion of findings assumes that responses at interview should be taken at face value. "Asians" claim to be too busy and have family commitments so, according to the report, they need motivating to prioritise screening for H pylori over other interests. However, the study offers no insights into how family members reach decisions. The authors give no details of the content or form of the written information so it is not possible to judge its motivational value or comprehensibility in either language. Being asked to give blood for purposes of research into an infection with a Latin name might understandably arouse suspicion or indifference in community members of any background. The fixed appointment time, the request for a reply slip (almost universally ignored), and the questions about demographic details all set a constrictive and even inquisitorial tone. With no personal contact with individuals, families or community leaders in support of the written word there would be no way that any doubts or fears about the purpose of the request could be allayed. Nevertheless, though seriously flawed, the study does indicate that far more than translation and posted letters and leaflets are needed to communicate with user groups on health issues in a way that is likely to be perceived as relevant and helpful.

Comparisons across studies

This study appears to corroborate the findings of earlier research (McAvoy and Raza, 1991) that postal materials are ineffective with minority ethnic users including those not fluent in English. However, there are possible confounding issues, including the extent to which the experimental design may actually distort decision making and subsequent health behaviour. Another issue is the assumption that a delivery mechanism (for example, a letter) may supply a solution to an issue ('non-compliance') which has been constructed entirely from a clinical viewpoint and without any prior research into user viewpoints and understandings. Appendix 4, Table 5 highlights some key comparisons between three health education materials and screening studies (McAvoy and Raza, 1991; Yancey et al, 1995; Stone et al, 1998).

EIGHT

Conclusions

Issues arising from the review

A picture emerges from the preceding chapters of persistent barriers that can only be dismantled if they are adequately conceptualised and recognised. Interpersonal processes of miscommunication arise from stereotyping, mismatching use and understanding of language, and mismatching beliefs and models of care. Workplace teams (for example, hospital wards and primary care practices), professional groups and user communities are all subject to differing socio-cultural influence. At the same time, these processes have been exacerbated by organisational problems in gathering and use of information about user communication needs, in provision of bilingual support and of material resources to meet identified need, and in practitioner education.

The interventions have achieved significant findings, with important implications for practice, although also leaving many issues unaddressed for research and development, and provision of services.

Among those findings, one area concerns the gathering and use of information about users' needs. It has been demonstrated that a feasible system for monitoring patient ethnicity and communication needs can be developed in primary care, to the satisfaction of practitioners (Monach and Davis, 1996). However, the issue remains of how a monitoring system can be effective in improving communications regarding patients' movements across different sectors of the health service. There is a need for further pilot studies concerning the way in which information is accessed and used across the NHS, and also for impact studies evaluating the effectiveness of monitoring in enhancing the quality of services. There is also a need for evaluation of staff training to assess and use information sensitively and effectively.

The issue of developing a service that is sensitive and responsive to cultural and ethnic diversity implicitly permeates all the communication interventions. However, specific micro-level interventions testing particular innovations such as videos for health education were more frequent than macro-level interventions evaluating the different qualities of entire services that were established to meet the needs of particular user groups. Among these groups are people with disabilities (for example, learning disabilities), older people and their families or carers, asylum seekers, people with specific conditions such as diabetes, and numerically dispersed minorities. Two studies (Snowden et al, 1995; Silove et al, 1997) evaluated aspects of specialist service development for minority ethnic patients in mental health, demonstrating that the culturally adapted specialist services, each marked by the presence of bilingual practitioners, among other factors, enhance satisfaction with aspects of communication and avoidance of unwanted emergency care.

Unfortunately, these studies fail to explore in any great depth what 'culturally sensitive' characteristics of the specialist service, in addition to the use of bilingual practitioners, account for their effectiveness and acceptability. The results imply that lessons can be learned for mainstream service development by involving user groups in examining in depth the different features of specialist services that contribute to user satisfaction.

Several interventions investigated the impact of bilingual services involving advocates, linkworkers, or interpreters, on a range of outcome measures including service use, user attitudes, and user health knowledge. One study (Parsons and Day, 1992) demonstrated significant effects of an antenatal advocacy service on obstetric outcomes, while leaving questions unanswered about the advocates' roles, and underlying that, models of provision. The use of bilingual advocates seems to be warranted by these findings as a means of improving maternal care. Yet there is a need for research which explores the range of roles bilingual health advocates might play, especially in their relations to health professionals, and to minority ethnic individual service users and communities. The tensions involved in such a range of roles for key participants need to be addressed. The meanings and limits of advocacy for those concerned need to be teased out and explored in relation to other key concepts in health policy, such as user empowerment. There is perhaps a need for future impact studies to be developed out of such research, rather than bypassing it.

Interventions assessing the impact of linkworkers on users' knowledge and use of health services have produced inconclusive results, both in relation to breast screening (Hoare et al, 1994), and maternal care (Mason, 1990). The reports of both studies beg questions about the roles of the linkworkers, leaving an impression that they were primarily supposed to supply health information, rather than undertake any of the more complex cultural brokerage roles requiring sensitivity to user needs and views (as discussed in Rocheron et al, 1989a, 1989b). That study lacks impact measures, but indicates that effective use of bilingual linkworkers requires attention to organisational factors such as adequate training for them and for clinical practitioners and independent line management, and improved employment conditions. The management team and practitioners need to be made sensitive to the work linkworkers can do in terms of accessing and facilitating user needs, as well as communicating health information or interpreting for practitioners. There is a need for research that combines a focus on the appropriate uses of linkworkers to maximise two-way communication between health professionals and minority ethnic service users, with a focus on measurable outcomes.

Several studies of interpreting services (for example Baker et al, 1996; Hornberger et al, 1996; Baker et al, 1998) taken together indicate that interpreting services with trained professional interpreters have a positive impact on a range of outcome measures (though the use of bilingual untrained professionals may have far fewer positive effects, while organisational weaknesses can seriously undermine services). For example, Hornberger et al (1996) found positive effects of a remote interpreting service intervention on user and professional satisfaction and communication process outcomes. But little attention is paid to cultural issues in interpreting, nor to professional concerns of the interpreter, and questions remain whether the outcomes had more to do with the 'distance' or the use of a simultaneous interpreting method. Baker et al (1998) found that untrained 'ad hoc' interpreters provide only a limited amount of patient interpersonal satisfaction. However, the definition of 'ad hoc' is itself vague and limited. In differing circumstances in primary or acute care, family members, or bilingual hospital staff, or even waiting room 'strangers', are used to act as interpreters. The reasons for using these different resources in different settings may vary contextually, and the impact of each on user and practitioner satisfaction or on effectiveness in terms of information transmission may vary too. Among the interventions carried out so far, the experimental designs, and predominantly quantitative approach to analysis, limit depth of insight into effects of interpreting services on communication across languages and cultures.

The existing studies provide consistent evidence that trained interpreters enhance communication. However, organisational and resource issues of implementing a practical service that meets both user demand and practitioner needs in all their variety remain to be addressed. To facilitate this, interventions comparing different methods of interpreting should be designed with more concern for transcultural communication than existing studies. Outcome measures are problematic if not grounded in the particular concerns of service users and professionals. A more far-reaching comparative approach may be required to investigate what relevant qualities trained interpreters bring to their work in comparison with different groups of 'untrained' interpreters. Such an approach would investigate closely what roles interpreters play in different communicative contexts. Qualitative attention also needs to be paid to cultural issues in interpreting, for example concerning confidentiality and user preferences.

The implementation of an effective policy-level intervention into bilingual service development depends greatly on structural and organisational aspects. Among such aspects are community consultation, effective service management in the context of equity and anti–racist issues, negotiation of aims and roles, sensitivity to local cultures and professional territorial concerns, commitment to quality training, and independent line management for bilingual workers. Yet such considerations have had little place in the reports of the relatively few impact studies which have been carried out.

Among several interventions concerned with communication training, two studies showed a positive impact of training clinical practitioners to work with interpreters on their use of interpreting services (Blackford et al, 1997; Stolk et al, 1998). At the same time, the Blackford study claims that the action research and training process made the nurses more reflective and more proactive in challenging inequities. Of course, the dilemma for any training programme is that its effectiveness will partly depend on the perceptions that practitioners have of service organisational flexibility, so that they can implement what they learn. One study showed a generally positive impact of a communication training module on medical students' communication skills (Farnill et al, 1997). Yet the study takes little account of user perspectives, and gives little consideration to what makes training culture sensitive.

One study found a positive impact of a receptionist training package on uptake of breast screening (Atri et al, 1997), although there are unanswered questions about the relative significance of the training and the language matching of receptionists with users. The importance of receptionists in primary and secondary care as gatekeepers to the health service is well recognised. Further research is needed to investigate the most effective ways of training receptionists to promote access. In practical terms, the most effective approaches may involve training that integrates receptionists with other members of health care teams, for example in primary care. Such an approach might, for example, focus on topics such as collecting and distributing information about patients' communication needs in order to anticipate and meet resource requirements. In this way, training becomes part of service development.

User involvement is a major issue underlying current models of service development. Yet it has been noted how rarely users are effectively involved in the development and implementation of research. One study trained local residents in Newcastle, UK, to research perceptions of psychological distress among Pakistani and Bangladeshi people in order to improve services (Kai and Hedges, 1999). The training and research resulted in subsequent initiatives from local services, principally recruitment of bilingual counsellors in non-general practice community settings, and a further programme of training in communication skills was started for local Asian people likely to encounter other peoples' distress. The model of counselling was adapted, a review of the NHS trust's mental health services for ethnic minorities was triggered, and local racism awareness training was prompted. This kind of research and training programme emphasising the challenges of user involvement has the potential of providing an evidence base for aligning service developments more closely with minority ethnic user group perceptions of need.

Finally, one report evaluates the impact of an interpreter training programme using a range of measures, including professional use of interpreting services (Farshi et al, 1999). The impact of interpreter training is diluted if it is not integrated with an effective, well-coordinated interpreting service development programme reaching all the sectors of the health service. This implies that management and practitioners may also require training, and that both organisational and attitudinal issues are paramount.

Interventions reviewed in the previous sections, though indicating positive effects of training, are vague about the content and processes of 'training packages'. Research is needed which builds on the current work but sets it in a context of institutional cultures and anti-racist awareness. There is also a need for research that pays close attention to the implications of language differences and cultural plurality on the details of training modules. Particular attention might be paid to areas of weakness for students – for example, for medical students, to adapting language to the hearer level and to facilitating emotional expression. The implications of researching the subject of transcultural communication for methodology and category development need careful assessment.

There is a lack of research evaluating programmes training professionals in skills of multi-party as well as two-way communication. Exploratory work is perhaps needed that focuses on different perceptions of roles, and underlying values and concerns in consultations among patients, relatives and community members, bilingual professionals and clinical professionals. A particular focus on training professionals to work with linkworkers might be beneficial.

One of the most productive methods of researching the effectiveness of communication skills training is the use of videotapes, or audio tapes with transcripts of interactions. Very little health research has pursued this option. In research into face-to-face interactions, there is a need for more refined use of categories of transcultural communicative skills. These would include, for example, both the communication of information and of interpersonal meanings, as well as responsive skills related to, for example, distribution of control over the topic of talk.

At a time when UK health service agendas prioritise inequalities (*Saving lives: Our healthier nation*, DoH, 1999a) and clinical governance (*Clinical governance*, DoH, 1999b), a desirable purpose of educational innovation would be to reduce discrepancies between academic theories of transcultural competence and communication, and the practitioners' 'theories in use' (Greenwood, 1993). Education for transcultural communication competence perhaps needs to engage more effectively with these processes, through observation and reflective practices. Better understandings are needed of the interaction between such theories in use, and the conditions of practice where attitudes and beliefs are nurtured. Such conditions might include presence of family members with patients during examinations, organisational issues concerning consultation time, and difficulties in obtaining and using interpreters. Such understandings require new research, which could contribute to the development of appropriate 'reflective' training methodologies in which the social and interpersonal complexities of transcultural communication in practice are given their due.

There appears to be a need for evaluated, post-registration training interventions with teams of practitioners working in localities having a substantial minority ethnic user population. One important direction concerns training professionals in skills of assessing users' communication needs and wants, and obtaining resources, as well as skills of communicating with and without bilingual professionals. Another direction (linked to the first) involves focusing on non-discriminatory communication practice. This might require looking at individual communication practice in relation to cultures and conditions in the workplace, and to effects at different levels. These levels might arguably include patient and practitioner understanding, satisfaction, empowerment, and proxy measures of improved care including service use. In fact, an aspect of evaluating training as a whole would be to assess its fit with, and consequences within, workplace environments.

In addition to the training of clinical professionals, research is needed which illuminates the organisational and cultural factors underlying service development in training and other areas. For example, the importance of managerial attitudes and awareness is recognised, especially with the current focus on mainstreaming cultural diversity and equity issues in the health service, but little research has focused on managers as change agents in relation to training priorities, or more generally, service development. The training of management may be a central plank of overall training programmes.

Finally, in this area, there is a need to link research on context-sensitive communication training to concerns about service development for transcultural communication. Such concerns might be met by an intervention focused on training a practice team, for example, in a haemoglobinopathy clinic or a diabetes clinic, to enhance communication. More generally, there is a need to develop context-sensitive research instruments for assessing the impact of training not only on individuals' awareness, attitudes and skills, but also on collective health service practice.

Among the interventions concerned with health education processes and materials, Brown et al (1996) demonstrated the positive impact of a community 'heart health' education programme involving bilingual group sessions and individual home-based work on minority ethnic service users' physical health. The emphasis on collective, culture-sensitive mediation of learning, and on sustained impact on a community, contrasts with the more limited individual outcome measures used elsewhere.

Several health education studies examined the impact of culturally sensitive materials on users' knowledge of health and health services, or their participation. Impact studies suggest that the combination of a 'culture sensitive video' or other culture sensitive materials, and aspects of 'person-to-person' contact, enhance outcomes such as screening or health knowledge. But the studies lack detailed consideration of the ways in which materials are to be developed and designated as culture sensitive. Each suffered from a lack of clarity about the influence of materials and of the methods used, and of the skills of practitioners delivering the education. In-depth qualitative approaches are needed to complement quantitative work and clarify these issues.

Nevertheless, clear gains were demonstrated for different interventions. For example, a pictorial education package in a one-to-one teaching programme led to improving diabetes knowledge, increased self-caring behaviour, and more positive attitudes to diabetes and the diabetes clinic (Hawthorne and Tomlinson, 1997). Yet the relative importance of pictorial materials, and one-to-one involvement with linkworkers is unclear, as flashcards alone would be ineffective. Two studies appeared to show that interventions involving the use of video to promote increased screening behaviour can be effective either in the home (McAvoy and Raza, 1991) or at a clinic waiting room (Yancey et al, 1995). Again, the effectiveness of home use of videos appeared to depend in part at least on the use of personal visits to promote their use, in comparison with the less effective method of sending postal information. More generally, the unanswered issues about which ingredients of health education strategies account for their relative success raise concerns about what constitutes culture sensitivity in research and service development as well as in the content of any communication intervention.

The lack of attention to important details about the format, content, language and style of the materials weakens most reports of such interventions. More evidence is required so that health professionals can, with confidence, develop and use materials, knowing that their form and content is proved to be effective for transcultural communication. The effectiveness of materials depends partly on how they are received. There is a need for studies that specifically focus on the participants' use and interpretation of materials in making decisions concerning their health. More generally, a recurrent concern for culture-sensitive service development and practice is that greater user involvement is required to meet user needs. In this way, not only might the concept of culture-sensitivity be clarified, for example in its relationship to ethnicity, in ways which enhance practice, but also other factors which might be neglected, such as age, class and gender sensitivity, may be brought forward.

Overall, the intervention findings summarised above illustrate the advantages of the primarily quantitative and quasi-experimental research approach that has held sway in providing a significant, although piecemeal evidence base for service development. At the same time, limitations have been noted for each group of studies, both in terms of the gaps in the research and in terms of the questions which remain unaddressed because of the rarity of much-needed impact studies which include qualitative methods. Implications arising from some of these limitations are summarised in the discussion further on.

Specific issues still need further clarification in order to provide a sound evidence base for service development recommendations. One area concerns consultation processes and assessment of user and provider needs in the development of services. The emphasis on user involvement in service development requires a greater corresponding emphasis in research on context-sensitive communications. Too little is known about the diverse socio-cultural contexts within which users' needs and values are felt and expressed, and which influence communications. Equally, there is a need for interventions that take greater account of the specific institutional contexts within which communications policy and practice are developed.

Related to the concern with consultations and needs assessment is the issue of how to evaluate interventions designed to enhance transcultural communication. Many interventions reviewed in this study are evaluated in terms of impact on individuals to some degree artificially abstracted from their social contexts. The challenge remains of re-contextualising work in this area in order to address questions of service development, and of equity of participation for specific user groups.

Many of the interventions hold out the encouraging promise that practical solutions to communication problems, such as the use of bilingual interpreters and culture-sensitive materials, will impact on various desirable outcomes in terms of service use, user and practitioner attitudes, or user health. Troublingly, however, few of the interventions seriously question what practitioner communication competencies in terms of skills, knowledge and attitudes are required to translate provision of resources into sustained transcultural and anti-racist practice. At the same time, there is a need for greater understanding of the impact on communication, for example, between nurses and minority ethnic patients, of major contextual and institutional influences on talk. Areas of importance are the impact of the workplace culture, of clinical tasks, of professional goals, of the presence of family members, and of divided attention on communication. A central concern is the impact of possibly mismatching expectations about health and service provision on communication. Such expectations may vary culturally and linguistically between health professionals and users.

Finally, research is needed to investigate models, processes and criteria for evaluating long-term effectiveness of health education programmes with individuals who are not fluent in English in their 'communities'. There is a need for greater clarity about underlying models of communication and care in this area. For example, the fit between cultural sensitivity and health service policy discourse highlighting user and practitioner empowerment (DoH, 2001a) needs careful exploration. Such issues link back to the initial concern with appropriate consultation mechanisms for cycles of research and development.

The evidence reviewed in this book offers hope for enhancing service development and practice in a wide range of areas. A concern remains whether the most appropriate research methods are being used to gain the evidence-based insights necessary to develop long-term strategies for effective communication in health services. The review strongly indicates that the development of effective strategies to overcome 'communication barriers' requires context-sensitive, needs-led initiatives. It also indicates that effective long-term strategies must address the interface between structural mechanisms and process aspects. For example, discriminatory practices such as shortcomings of language provision and instances of racist stereotyping can be understood as effects of organisational failures of service management and training, but also as effects of collectively mediated attitudes and of inadequacies of transcultural communication skills among health professionals. The development of an appropriate knowledge base to underpin service development requires approaches sensitive to the dynamics of structure and process. It also requires sensitivity to the changing and heterogeneous environments of the health service and of diverse minority ethnic groups, where some users continue to experience urgent difficulties connected to communication in accessing and using the health service.

References

Ahmad, W. (ed) (1993) *'Race' and health in contemporary Britain*, Buckingham: Open University Press.

Ahmad, W. (1993) 'Making black people sick: 'race', ideology and health research', in W. Ahmad (ed) *'Race' and health in contemporary Britain*, Buckingham: Open University Press, pp 11–33.

Ahmad, W. (1996) 'The trouble with culture', in D. Kelleher and S. Hillier (eds) *Researching cultural differences in health*, London: Routledge, pp 190–219.

Ahmad, W. and Walker, R. (1997) *Asian older people: Housing, health and access to services*, Bradford: Ethnicity and Social Policy Research Unit, Department of Social and Economic Studies, University of Bradford.

Ahmad, W., Kernohan, E and Baker, M. (1991) 'Patients' choice of general practitioner: Patients' and doctors' sex and ethnicity', *British Journal of General Practice*, vol 41, no 349, pp 330–1.

Annandale, E. (1999) *The sociology of health and medicine*, Cambridge: Polity Press.

Anderson, J., Wiggins, S., Rajwani, R., Holbrook, A., Blue, C. and Ng, M. (1995) 'Living with a chronic illness: Chinese-Canadian and Euro-Canadian women with diabetes – exploring factors that influence management', *Social Science & Medicine*, vol 41, no 2, pp 181-95.

Arai, Y. and Farrow, S. (1995) 'Access, expectations and communication: Japanese mothers' interaction with GPs in a pilot study in North London', *Public Health*, vol 109, no 5, pp 353-61.

Arora, R. (ed); Husband, C., Singh, M. and Slevin, M. and the University of Bradford Race Relations Research Unit and Bradford and Ilkley Community College (1995) *The language needs assessment project: Report of a research project funded by the Patients Charter*, Race Relations Research Unit, and Bradford Community Health NHS Trust.

Atkinson, P. (1995) *Medical talk and medical work: The liturgy of the clinic*, London: Sage Publications.

Atri, J., Falshaw, M., Gregg, R., Robson, J., Omar, R. and Dixon, S. (1997) 'Improving uptake of breast screening in multiethnic populations: a randomised controlled trial using practice reception staff to contact non-attenders', *British Medical Journal*, vol 315, pp 1356-9.

Bahl, V. (1988) *The employment and training of linkworkers: A report of the work carried out in the pilot districts in the Asian mother and baby campaign*, London: Department of Health and Social Security.

Baker, D., Hayes, R. and Fortier, J. (1998) 'Interpreter use and satisfaction with interpersonal aspects of care for Spanish-speaking patients', *Medical Care*, vol 36, no 10, pp 1461-70.

Baker, D., Parker, R., Williams, M., Coates, W. and Pitkin, K. (1996) 'Use and effectiveness of interpreters in an emergency department', *JAMA*, vol 275, no 10, pp 783-8.

Baker, E., Bouldin, N., Durham, M., Lowell, M., Gonzales, M., Jodaitis, N., Cruz, L., Torres, I., Torres, M. and Adams, S. (1997) 'The Latino Health Advisory Program: a collaborative lay health advisor approach', *Health Education and Behaviour*, vol 24, no 4, pp 495-509.

Barker, P. (2000) 'Reflections on caring as a virtue ethic within an evidence-based culture', *International Journal of Nursing Studies*, vol 37, pp 329-36.

Baxter, C. (1993) *The communication needs of black and ethnic minority pregnant women in Salford: A report on a needs assessment exercise*, Salford: Salford Health Authority.

Baxter, C., Baylav, A., Fuller, J., Marr, A and Sanders, M. (1996) *The case for the provision of bilingual services within the NHS*, London: Bilingual Health Advocacy Project, and Department of Health.

Bhatt, A. and Dickinson, R. (1993) *Evaluation of health education materials for ethnic minorities: A research project funded by the Department of Health: Final report*, Leicester: University of Leicester Centre for Mass Communication Research, and Department of Health.

Bhatti-Sinclair, K. and Wheal, A. (1998a) 'Using external audit to review ethnically sensitive practice', *Journal of Clinical Effectiveness*, vol 3, no 1, pp 2-5.

Bhatti-Sinclair, K. and Wheal, A. (1998b) 'Analysis of the external audit on ethnically sensitive practice', *Journal of Clinical Effectiveness*, vol 3, no 1, pp 6-9.

Blackford, J., Street, A. and Parsons, C. (1997) 'Breaking down language barriers in clinical practice', *Contemporary Nurse*, vol 6, no 1, pp 15-21.

Bowes, A. and Domokos, T. (1995a) 'South Asian women and their GPs: Some issues of communication', *Social Sciences in Health: International Journal of Research & Practice*, vol 1, no 1, pp 22-33.

Bowes, A. and Domokos, T. (1995b) 'Key issues in South Asian women's health: A study in Glasgow', *Social Sciences in Health: International Journal of Research & Practice*, vol 1, no 3, pp 145-57.

Bowler, I.M.W. (1993) 'Stereotypes of women of Asian descent in midwifery: Some evidence', *Midwifery*, vol 9, no 1, pp 7-16.

Box, V. (1998) 'Cervical screening: the knowledge and opinions of black and minority ethnic women and of health advocates in East London', *Health Education Journal,* vol 57, no 1, pp 3-15.

Brown, P. and Levinson, S. (1987) *Politeness*, Cambridge: Cambridge University Press.

Brown, W., Lee, C. and Oyomopito, R. (1996) 'Effectiveness of a bilingual heart health program for Greek-Australian women', *Health Promotion International*, vol 11, no 2, pp 117-25.

Buckinghamshire Health Authority (1996) *Communicating with our ethnic minority communities: How should we do it? A survey of good practice, practical experience and community ideas*, Aylesbury: ACCPK consultants.

Burton, A. (2000) 'Reflection: Nursing's practice and education panacea?', *Journal of Advanced Nursing*, vol 31, no 5, pp 1009-17.

Cameron, R. and Williams, J. (1997) 'Sentence to ten cents: A case study of relevance and communicative success in nonnative-native speaker interactions in a medical setting', *Applied Linguistics*, vol 18, no 4, pp 415-45.

Centre for Public Policy and Urban Change (1999) *An integrated communication strategy for Birmingham*, Birmingham: University of Central England.

Chahal, K. (1996) *Minority ethnic health in Crawley*, Crawley: West Sussex Health Authorities.

Chu, C. (1998) 'Cross-cultural health issues in contemporary Australia', *Ethnicity & Health*, vol 3, no 1-2, pp 125-34.

Clevely Northgate Trust (1987) *The role of an Asian advocate with the health services.*

Coupland, N. and Coupland J. (1998) 'Reshaping lives: constitutive identity work in geriatric medical consultations', *Text*, vol 18, no 2, pp 159-89.

Coupland, N., Giles, H. and Wiemann, J. (eds) (1991) *'Miscommunication' and problematic talk*, London:Sage.

Coupland, N. and Jaworski, A. (1997) 'Relevance, accommodation and conversation: modeling the social dimension of communication', *Multilingua*, vol 16, nos 2/3, pp 233-58.

Crystal, D. (1987) *The Cambridge encylopedia of language*, Cambridge: Cambridge University Press.

Culley, L. (1996) 'A critique of multiculturalism in health care: the challenge for nurse education', *Journal of Advanced Nursing*, vol 23, pp 564-70.

DoH (Department of Health) (1999a) *Saving lives: Our healthier nation*, Cm 4386, Norwich:The Stationery Office.

DoH (1999b) *Clinical governance: In the new NHS*, HSC 065, Health service circular.

DoH (1999c) *Making a difference: Strengthening the nursing, midwifery and health visiting contribution to health and healthcare*, Norwich:The Stationery Office.

DoH (2000) *The vital connection: An equalities framework for the NHS*, Norwich:The Stationery Office.

DoH (2001) *Race equality in the Department of Health: The Race Relations (Amendment) Act 2000*, Norwich:The Stationery Office.

DoH (2001a) *Shifting the balance of power within the NHS, securing delivery*, Norwich:The Stationery Office.

DoH (2001b) *The expert patient:A new approach to chronic disease management for the 21st century*, Norwich:The Stationery Office.

Dowse, R. and Ehlers, M. (1998) 'Pictograms in pharmacy', *The International Journal of Pharmacy Practice*, vol 6, pp 109-118.

Drew, P. and Heritage, J. (eds) (1992) *Talk at work*, Cambridge: Cambridge University Press.

Elder, J., Candelaria, J., Woodruff, S., Golbeck, A., Criqui, M., Talavera, G., Rupp, J. and Domier, C. (1998) 'Initial results of "Language for Health": Cardiovascular disease nutrition education for English-as-a-second-language students', *Health Education Research*, vol 13, no 4, pp 567-75.

Farnill, D., Todisco, J., Hayes, S. and Bartlett, D. (1997) 'Videotaped interviewing of non-English speakers: training for medical students with volunteer clients', *Medical Education*, vol 31, no 2, pp 87-93.

Farooq, S., Fear, C. and Oyebode, F. (1997) 'An investigation of the adequacy of psychiatric interviews conducted through an interpreter', *Psychiatric Bulletin*, vol 21, no 4, pp 209-13.

Farshi, Z., Atkinson K. and Sleight J. (1999) *Evaluation of the Leeds NHS interpreting project*, Leeds: The Leeds Teaching Hospitals NHS Trust.

Fenton, S. and Sadiq Sangster, A. (1996) 'Culture, relativism and the expression of mental distress: South Asian women in Britain', *Sociology of Health and Illness*, vol 18, no 1, pp 66-85.

Free, C., White, P., Shipman, C. and Dale, J. (1999) 'Access to and use of out-of-hours services by members of Vietnamese community groups in South London: A focus group study', *Family Practice* vol 16, no 4, pp 369-74.

Freud, S. (1936) *The ego and mechanisms of defence*, London: Chatto and Windus.

Gerrish, K. (2000) 'Individual care: its conceptualisation and practice within a multi-ethnic society', *Journal of Advanced Nursing*, vol 32, no 1, pp 91-9.

Gerrish, K. (2001) 'The nature and effect of communication difficulties arising from interactions between district nurses and South Asian patients and their carers', *Journal of Advanced Nursing*, vol 33, no 5, pp 566-74.

Gerrish, K. Husband, C. and Mackenzie, J. (1996) *Nursing for a multi-ethnic society*, Buckingham: Open University Press.

Goffman, E. (1981) *Forms of talk*, Oxford: Blackwell.

Good, B. and Good, M. (1994) 'In the subjunctive mode: Epilepsy narratives in Turkey', *Social Science and Medicine*, vol 38, pp 835-42.

Greenwood, J. (1993) 'Reflective practice: A critique of the work of Argyris and Schon', *Journal of Advanced Nursing*, vol 18, pp 1183-97.

Guarnaccia, P. and Rodriguez, O. (1996) 'Concepts of culture and their role in the development of culturally competent mental health services', *Hispanic Journal of Behavioral Sciences*, vol 18, no 4, pp 419-43.

Gudykunst, W. and Kim, Y. (1992a) *Communicating with strangers*, New York, NY: McGraw Hill.

Gudykunst, W. and Kim, Y. (eds) (1992b) *Readings on communicating with strangers*, New York, NY: McGraw Hill.

Gumperz, J. (1992) *Discourse strategies*, Cambridge: Cambridge University Press.

Hasselkus, B. (1992) 'The family caregiver as interpreter in the geriatric medical interview', *Medical Anthropology Quarterly*, vol 6, no 3, pp 288-304.

Hatton, C., Azmi, S., Caine, A. and Emerson, E. (1998) 'Informal carers of adolescents and adults with learning difficulties from the South Asian communities: family circumstances, service support and carer stress', *British Journal of Social Work*, vol 28, no 6, pp 821-37.

Hatton, D. and Webb, T. (1993) 'Information transmission in bilingual, bicultural contexts: A field study of community health nurses and interpreters', *Journal of Community Health Nursing*, vol 10, no 3, pp 137-47.

Hawthorne, K. and Tomlinson, S. (1997) 'One-to-one teaching with pictures: Flashcard health education for British Asians with diabetes', *British Journal of General Practice*, vol 47, no 418, pp 301-4.

Heritage, J. and Sefi, S. (1992) 'Dilemmas of advice: aspects of the delivery and reception of advice in interactions between health visitors and first time mothers', in P. Drew and J. Heritage (eds) pp 359-417.

Hillier, S. and Kelleher, D. (1996) 'Considering culture, ethnicity and the politics of health', in D. Kelleher and S. Hillier (eds) *Researching cultural differences in health*, London: Routledge pp 1-10.

Hoare, T., Thomas, C., Biggs, A., Booth, M., Diadley, S. and Friedman, F. (1994) 'Can the uptake of breast screening by Asian women be increased? A randomized controlled trial of a linkworker intervention', *Journal of Public Health Medicine*, vol 16, no 2, pp179-85.

Hornberger, J., Gibson, C., Wood, W., Dequeldre, C., Corso, I., Palla, B. and Bloch, D. (1996) 'Eliminating language barriers for non-English-speaking patients', *Medical Care*, vol 34, no 8, pp 845-56.

Hyden L-C. and Mishler, E. (1999) 'Language and medicine', *Annual Review of Applied Linguistics*, vol 19, pp 174-92.

Ilett. S. (1995) 'Putting it on tape: Audio taped assessment summaries for parents', *Archives of Disease in Childhood*, vol 73, no 5, pp 435-8.

Jaggi, A. and Bithell, C. (1995) 'Relationships between physiotherapists' level of contact, cultural awareness and communication with Bangladeshi patients in two health authorities', *Physiotherapy*, vol 81, no 6, pp 330-7.

Jaworski, A. and Coupland, N. (eds) (1997) *The discourse reader*, London: Routledge.

Johnson, K. (1996) *Language teaching and skill learning*, Oxford: Blackwell.

Johnson, M. (1996) 'Ethnic minorities, health and communication', Research Paper in *Ethnic Relations*, no 24, Leicester: University of Leicester.

Kai, J. and Hedges, C. (1999) 'Minority ethnic community participation in needs assessment and service development in primary care: Perceptions of Pakistani and Bangladeshi people about psychological distress', *Health Expectations*, vol 2, pp 7-20.

Karim, J. (1996) *Access to accident and emergency services for minority ethnic residents*, Birmingham: Birmingham Heartlands and Solihull NHS Trust (Teaching).

Kelleher, D. (1996) 'A defence of "ethnicity" and "culture"', in D. Kelleher and S. Hillier (eds) *Researching cultural differences in health*, London: Routledge, pp 69-90.

Kelleher, D. and Hillier, S. (eds) (1996) *Researching cultural differences in health*, London: Routledge.

Kim, Y. (1992) 'Intercultural communication competence: a systems theoretic view', in W. Gudykunst and Y. Kim (eds) *Readings on communicating with strangers*, New York, NY: McGraw Hill.

Kurtz, S., Silverman, J. and Draper, J. (eds) (1998) *Teaching and learning communication skills in medicine*, Oxford: Radcliffe Medical Press.

Lam, T. and Green, J. (1994) 'Primary health care and the Vietnamese community: A survey in Greenwich', *Health & Social Care in the Community*, vol 2, no 5, pp 293-9.

Lambert, H. and Sivak, L. (1996) 'Is "cultural difference" a useful concept? Perceptions of health and the sources of ill health among Londoners of South Asian origin', in D.Kelleher and S.Hillier (eds) *Researching cultural differences in health*, London: Routledge, pp 124-59.

Law, I. (1996) *Racism, ethnicity and social policy*, Hemel Hempstead: Prentice Hall.

Lawrenson, R., Leydon, G., Freeman, G., Fuller, J., Ballard, J. and Ineichen, B. (1998) 'Are we providing for ethnic diversity in accident & emergency (A&E) departments?', *Ethnicity & Health*, vol 3, nos 1/2, pp117-23.

Leather, C., Wirz, S. and Hook, E. (1996) *The training and development needs of bilingual support workers in the NHS in community settings*, London: Centre for International Child Health and Department of Health, NHS Executive.

Leets, L., Giles, H. and Clement, R. (1996) 'Explicating ethnicity in theory and communication research', *Multilingua*, vol 15, no 2, pp 115-47.

Leininger, M. (1984) 'Transcultural nursing: an essential knowledge and practice field for today', *Canadian Nurse*, December, pp 41-57.

Lemmer, B., Grellier, R. and Steven, J. (1999) 'Systematic review of non-random and qualitative research literature: Exploring and uncovering an evidence base for health visiting and decision making', *Qualitative Health Research*, vol 9, no 3, pp 315-18.

Levenson, R. and Gillam, S. (1998) *Linkworkers in primary care*, London: The King's Fund.

Lupton, D. (1994) 'Toward the development of critical health communication praxis', *Health Communication*, vol 6, no 1, pp 55-67.

McAvoy, B. and Raza, R. (1988) 'Asian women: 1, Contraceptive knowledge, attitudes and usage. 2, Contraceptive services and cervical cytology', *Health Trends*, no 20, pp 11-16.

McAvoy, B. and Raza, R. (1991) 'Can health education increase uptake of cervical smear testing among Asian women?', *British Medical Journal*, vol 302, pp 833-6.

MacDonald, R. (1998) 'What is cultural competency?', *British Journal of Occupational Therapy*, vol 61, no 7, pp 325-28.

McNamara, B., Martin, K., Waddell, C. and Yuen, K. (1997) 'Palliative care in a multicultural society: Perceptions of health care professionals', *Palliative Medicine*, vol 11, no 5, pp 359-67.

MacPherson Report (1999) *The Stephen Lawrence inquiry: Report of an inquiry by Sir William MacPherson of Cluny*, Cm 4262-1, London: Home Office.

McTear, M. and King, F. (1991) 'Miscommunication in clinical contexts: The speech therapy interview', in N. Coupland, H. Giles and J. Wiemann (eds) *'Miscommunication' and problematic talk*, London: Sage, pp 195-214.

Martin, J. and Nakayama, T. (1999) 'Thinking dialectically about culture and communication', *Communication Theory*, vol 9, no 1, pp 1-25.

Mason, E., (1990) 'The Asian mother and baby campaign (the Leicestershire experience)', *Journal of the Royal Society of Health*, vol 110, no 1, pp 1-4, 9.

Maynard, D. (1992) 'On clinicians co-implicating recipients' perspective in the delivery of diagnostic news', in P. Drew and J. Heritage (eds) *Talk at work*, Cambridge: Cambridge University Press, pp 331-58.

Mays, N. and Pope, C. (1995) 'Rigour and qualitative research', *British Medical Journal*, vol 311, pp 109-12.

Miles, R. (1989) *Racism*, London: Routledge.

Mitchell, P., Malak, A. and Small, D. (1998) 'Bilingual professionals in community mental health services', *Australian and New Zealand Journal of Psychiatry*, vol 32, no 3, pp 424-33.

Monach, J. and Davis S. (1996) *Primary care ethnic monitoring pilot project*, Sheffield: Sheffield Centre for Health and Related Research, University of Sheffield.

Murphy, K. and Macleod Clark, J. (1993) 'Nurses' experiences of caring for ethnic-minority clients', *Journal of Advanced Nursing*, vol 18, no 3, pp 442-50.

Naish, J., Brown, J. and Denton, B. (1994) 'Intercultural consultations: Investigation of factors that deter non-English-speaking women from attending their general practitioners for cervical screening', *British Medical Journal*, vol 309, pp 1126-8.

Nazroo, J. (1998) 'Genetic cultural or socio-economic vulnerability? Explaining ethnic inequalities in health', *Sociology of Health and Illness*, vol 20, no 5, pp 710-30.

Newman, M. (1999) (unpublished) *;Evidence-based nursing tutors' critical appraisal manual*, School of HeBES, Middlesex University.

Papadopoulos, I. and Alleyne, J. (1998) 'Health of minority ethnic groups' in I.Papadopoulos, M.Tilki and J.Alleyne (eds) *Transcultural care:A guide for health care professionals*, Dinton: Mark Allen pp 1-17.

Papadopoulos, I., Tilki, M. and Alleyne, J. (1998) *Transcultural care:A guide for health care professionals*, Dinton: Mark Allen.

Parsons, L. and Day, S. (1992) 'Improving obstetric outcomes in ethnic minorities – an evaluation of health advocacy in Hackney', *Journal of Public Health Medicine*, vol 14, no 2, pp 183-91.

Pauwels, A. (1990) 'Health professionals' perceptions of communication difficulties in cross-cultural contexts', *Australian Review of Applied Linguistics*, Supplement 7, pp 93-111.

Pendleton, D. and Hasler, J. (eds) (1983) *Doctor-patient communication*, London: Academic Press.

Perakyla, A. (1998) 'Authority and accountability: The delivery of diagnosis in primary health care', *Social Psychology Quarterly*, vol 61, no 4, pp 301-20.

Phipps, D. (1995) 'Occupational therapy practice with clients from non-English speaking backgrounds: A survey of clinicians in south-west Sydney', *Australian Occupational Therapy Journal*, vol 42, no 4, pp 151-60.

Platzer, H., Blake, D. and Ashford, D. (2000) 'An evaluation of process and outcomes from learning through reflective practice groups on a post-registration nursing course', *Journal of Advanced Nursing*, vol 31, no 3, pp. 689-95.

Plunkett, A. and Quine, S. (1996) 'Difficulties experienced by carers from non-English-speaking backgrounds in using health and other support services', *Australian and New Zealand Journal of Public Health*, vol 20, no 1, pp 27-32.

Podro, S. (1994) *Training in bilingual advocacy: The British, Belgian and French experience of intercultural mediation*, London: Interpreting Project.

Popay, J., Rogers, A. and Williams, G. (1998) 'Rationale and standards for the systematic review of qualitative literature in health services research', *Qualitative Health Research*, vol 8, no 3, pp 341-51.

Rehbein, J. (1994) 'Rejective proposals: Semi-professional speech and clients' varieties in intercultural doctor-patient communication', *Multilingua*, vol 13, no 12, pp 83-130.

Rich, A. and Parker, D. (1995) 'Reflection and critical incident analysis: ethical and moral implications of their use within nursing and midwifery education', *Journal of Advanced Nursing*, vol 22, pp 1050-57.

Ritch, A., Ehtisham, M., Guthrie, S., Talbot, J., Luck, M. and Tinsley, R. (1996) 'Ethnic influences on health and dependency of elderly inner city residents', *Journal of the Royal College of Physicians of London*, vol 30, no 3, pp 215-20.

Roberts, C. (1998) 'Awareness in intercultural communication', *Language Awareness*, vol 7, pp 109-27.

Robinson, L. (1998) '*Race*', *communication and the caring professions*, Buckingham: Open University Press.

Rocheron, Y., Dickinson, R. and Khan, S. (1989a) *Evaluation of Asian mother and baby campaign: Full summary report*, Leicester: Centre for Mass Communication Research, University of Leicester.

Rocheron, Y., Khan, S. and Dickinson, R. (1989b) 'Links across a divide', *Health Service Journal*, vol 99, pp 951-2.

Rodwell, C. (1996) 'An analysis of the concept of empowerment', *Journal of Advanced Nursing*, vol 23, pp 305-13.

Roter, D. and Hall, J. (1989) 'Studies of doctor–patient interaction', *Annual Review of Public Health*, vol 10, pp 163-80.

Saldov, M. and Chow, P. (1994) 'The ethnic elderly in Metro Toronto hospitals, nursing-homes, and homes for the aged', *Communication and Health Care*, vol 38, no 2, pp 117-35.

Sarangi, S. (1994) 'Intercultural or not? Beyond celebration of cultural differences in miscommunication analysis', *Pragmatics*, vol 4, no 3, pp 409-27.

Scollon, R. and Scollon, S. (1995) *Intercultural Communication*, Oxford: Blackwell.

Shah, R. (1997) 'Improving services to Asian families and children with disabilities', *Child: Care, Health & Development*, vol 23, no 1, pp 41-6.

Shah, R. and Piracha, A. (1993) *Hello can you here me? A study of the communication experiences of the Asian community with health services in Blackburn, Hyndburn and Ribble Valley Health Authority*, Blackburn, Hyndburn and Ribble Valley Health Authority, Health Promotion Unit.

Shea, A. (1997) *Somali link-worker project evaluation report*, White City Health Centre, Hammersmith, Riverside Community Health Care Trust, and Somali Caring and Education Association, Fulham.

Silove, D., Manicavasagar, V., Beltran, R., Le, G., Nguyen, H., Phan, T. and Blaszczynski, A. (1997) 'Satisfaction of Vietnamese patients and their families with refugee and mainstream mental health services', *Psychiatric Services*, vol 48, no 8, pp 1064-69.

Silverman, D. (1987) *Communication and medical practice: Social relations in the clinic*, London: Sage.

Smaje, C. (1995) *Health, 'race' and ethnicity: Making sense of the evidence*, London: King's Fund Institute.

Smaje, C. (1996) 'The ethnic patterning of health: New directions for theory and research', *Sociology of Health and Illness*, vol 18, no 2, pp 141-71.

Small, R., Rice, P., Yelland, J. and Lumley, J. (1999) 'Mothers in a new country: The role of culture and communication in Vietnamese, Turkish and Filipino women's experiences of giving birth in Australia', *Women & Health*, vol 28, no 3, pp 77-101.

Snowden, L., Hu, T.W. and Jerrell, J. (1995) 'Emergency care avoidance: Ethnic matching and participation in minority-serving programs', *Community Mental Health Journal*, vol 31, no 5, pp 463-73.

Sourial, S. (1997) 'An analysis of caring', *Journal of Advanced Nursing*, vol 26, no 6, pp 1189-92.

Stephenson, P. (1995) 'Vietnamese refugees in Victoria, B.C. An overview of immigrant and refugee health care in a medium-sized Canadian urban centre', *Social Science & Medicine*, vol 40, no 12, pp 1631-42.

Stolk, Y. Ziguras, S. Saunders, T. Garlick, R. Stuart, G. and Coffey, G. (1998) 'Lowering the language barrier in an acute psychiatric setting', *Australian and New Zealand Journal of Psychiatry*, vol 32, no 3, pp 434-40.

Stone, M. Patel, H. Panja, K. Barnett, D. and Mayberry, J. (1998) 'Reasons for non-compliance with screening for infection with Helicobacter pylori, in a multi-ethnic community in Leicester, UK', *Public Health*, vol 112, no 3, pp 153-6.

Trill, M. and Holland, J. (1993) 'Cross-cultural differences in the care of patients with cancer: A review', *General Hospital Psychiatry*, vol 15, no 1, pp 21-30.

Trinh, Q. (1996) *Final report: Maternity development project for the Vietnamese community in Deptford and Lewisham*, Maternity Development Project for Vietnamese Community.

Vydelingum, V. (2000) 'South Asian patients' lived experience of acute care in an English hospital', *Journal of Advanced Nursing*, vol 32, no 1, pp 100-7.

Warrier, S. and Goodman, M. (eds) (1996) 'Consumer empowerment: A qualitative study of linkworker and advocacy services for non-English speaking users of maternity services, executive summary', The Maternity Alliance.

Yancey, A., Tanjasiri, S., Klein, M. and Tunder, J. (1995) 'Increased cancer screening behavior in women of color by culturally sensitive video exposure', *Preventive Medicine*, vol 24, no 2, pp 142-8.

Appendix I: Protocol extracts

Objectives

A. To review the main conceptual frameworks used in empirical research into communication between minority ethnic health care users who may not be fluent in English and service providers.
B. To identify (from English language literature) barriers to communication that may influence access and participation in health care for adult health care users who may not be fluent in English.
C. To identify recommended practices which, if implemented, might overcome barriers to communication and enhance communication.

Interventions

D. To identify and describe (from English language literature) interventions which have been implemented to enhance communication/overcome barriers affecting communication between adult health care users who may not be fluent in English and service providers.
E. To evaluate the effectiveness of any such interventions in terms of measured outcomes.
F. To evaluate the range of outcome measures used in intervention studies.
G. To evaluate the studies against a range of criteria for credibility and transferability.
H. To evaluate studies against 'barriers' that have been identified.
I. To identify key considerations for service development and research.

Types of study – criteria for inclusion

The empirical part of the review as opposed to the conceptual part describes:

either:

> studies designed to assess or illuminate barriers to communication as these may impact on access and participation;

or:

> studies describing interventions designed to overcome barriers and enhance communication with adult health care users who may not be fluent in English.

Studies are data based. Interventions selected are all evaluated by the intervention report authors, rather than only described.

Design types may include:

> quasi–experimental, comparative studies;

or:

> developmental, comparative or non–comparative studies.

Among key considerations for inclusion of empirical barrier or intervention studies, necessary criteria are:

- Participants: the study should indicate its relevance to adult minority ethnic health care users who lack fluency in English.
- Setting: the relevance of the setting to communication between adult health care users who lack fluency in English and service providers should be indicated.
- Aims: the study should aim to identify barriers to communication or to enhance communication between adult health care users who lack fluency in English and service providers.
- Outcomes: there should be empirical outcomes, related to the aims, reported in the study.

The main reason for limiting the number of necessary criteria is that too narrow a range for the review would drastically reduce its potential to provide a potent analysis of communication issues. Such issues concern not just face-to-face communication processes but also structural factors..

Description and evaluation of selected studies

An extraction form was developed primarily as a device for structured and comparative description but there is also scope for evaluation. Principles and guidelines for the comparative evaluation of studies are set out in the extraction form in Appendix 2.

Search terms

The search terms and strategies used necessarily varied for different databases. Nevertheless, a number of key terms or their available permutations, abbreviations and indexed synonyms were used in the different databases. These are: communication; communication barriers; communication skills; access; racism; culture or cross-cultural or intercultural; ethnic; minority groups; interpreter or interpreting services; intervention or intervention studies; controlled studies/trials; evaluation studies; language; advocacy; linkworker.

Where possible, indexing terms and free text terms were both used. A sample search is shown in Appendix 3.

The following databases were used: Medline, Embase, Cinahl, Cochrane library databases, HMIC DH database, HMIC King's Fund, PsychLIT, Social Science Citation Index, Sociofile, Sociological Abstracts, ERIC, British Education Index, Linguistic and Language Behaviour Abstracts (Cambridge Scientific Abstracts), Dissertation Abstracts, CRIB.

The search for 'grey' literature also extended to the use of NHS Ethnic Health Unit bibliographies, and contacts with Health Authorities. In such a wide field as communication in health care it is unlikely that the search, though carefully structured, could be exhaustive.

Appendix 2: Data extraction form

Part 1: Description of study

Study

Reviewer

Bibliographic details

Research question and aims

Is there a statement of the aims of the study?

Study methodology

Study type: (eg evaluation of barriers, intervention study)

Study design:
    (barrier study or intervention study)
    (developmental)
    (experimental)
    (is the study comparison or non–comparison?)

How were participants in the study recruited or selected?

What are the level(s) and type(s) of the barriers identified?
    (levels may include: structural, communication processes, both)

What, if any, type and level of recommendations for interventions are made?

What, if any, are the level(s), type(s), and content of the intervention?

Which of the following outcome measures were used in the intervention study? (add detail):
a. measures of structural/organizational practice
b. measures of communication patterns/processes
c. measures of attitude or belief or knowledge
d. assessments of health/well-being
e. measures of frequency of use/patterns of use of service
f. other

How was data collected? By what methods; from whom; and where?

When was the study, and when was data collected?

Settings

In which country, which broad area of health practice, and which region did the study take place?

Participants

Who were the co-participants? (expand where possible with age, gender, ethnicity, socio-economic status)

Where were barriers identified, and where did the intervention take place?

Who was identified as the target group and the specific 'recipients' of any intervention (eg Spanish-speaking users receive interpreter)?

What was the number of participants in any/each intervention group?

Evaluation of barriers only

How was the study developed (eg processes through which it came about)?

What was the length of the study?

What type of evidence is offered?

Intervention studies only

Name of intervention (if any)?

How was the intervention developed?

What rationale is given for the intervention?

What was the length and frequency of the intervention?

Who provided the intervention?

What resources were required for the intervention (eg training of providers, material resources)?

Results or findings

Interpretations of findings

Conducted by author

Part 2: Assessment of quality of studies

A: Non-experimental/developmental study

(Note if standard of reporting affects evaluation of methodology)

Are aims clear?

Have key parties been consulted in development of research and communication of findings?

Is research methodology explicit and matched to aims (are key constructs operationalised with clarity and sufficient to purpose)?

Is information on sample systematic, eg sufficient and appropriate to the aims and methodology, with a rationale for sample selection?

Is design and method of data collection described in sufficient detail, appropriate to aims, and dependable, with rationale provided?

Are multiple methods and sources of collection used?

If interviews are used, are interview questions shown, pre-tested, and refined progressively?

Are interviews recorded and transcribed?

If observation is used is due attention paid to influence of context?

Are methods of analysis of data described in sufficient and systematic detail? Are categories and measures adequate to aims?

Is use made of any exceptional cases?

Is analysis handled or assessed by more than one person? Do participants contribute?

Is analysis strengthened by counting of instances?

Is 'context' a resource for the study or are its effects under-analysed?

How is attention paid to the description and interpretation of subjective meanings and of lay knowledge?

Is the statement of findings clear? (see Part 1). Do the findings match aims and measures?

Credibility/reliability

Were efforts made to assess credibility/reliability through the following:

Detailed recording of data and process of analysis?

Use of methods that are feasible to replicate?

Use of any inter-rater reliability methods?

Plausibility/transferability/validity

Were efforts made to assess validity through the following:

Is the study generalised in terms of theories?

Is there comparative and contrastive use of multiple methods and sources for data collection and analysis?

Is there participant evaluation to compare with researchers' explanations?

Is there comparison of population with larger samples/coordination of studies?

Is there recognition of exception/inconsistencies in results?

Interpretations of findings from data (see Part 1)

Are interpretations of results presented clearly with sufficient data analysis, and presented distinctly from descriptions of settings, report of results, and report of viewpoints?

Are the interventions or the developmental studies evaluated?

Are selected omissions from data-set (eg parts of transcripts) accounted for adequately?

How adequate is the offered explanation to the problem and to other evidence?

Are alternative interpretations considered?

Is the context sufficiently considered, to support interpretations?

Are implications discussed in terms of:
a. addressing research aim?
b. suggesting further research?
c. impacting on policy/practice?
d. contribution to theory development/understanding in relation to other work?
e. applicability to different populations/contexts/settings?

Has there been critical examination of possible sources of bias, eg through separate treatment of data, analytic framework, interpretation?

Are findings credible and transferable?

Are findings useful for:
a. illuminating barriers?
b   identifying interventions?
c. evaluating interventions?

B: Experimental/controlled study

(Note if standard of reporting affects evaluation of methodology)

Are research aims clear?

Have key participants or interested parties been consulted in development of research and communication of findings?

Is intervention type explained adequately in terms of issue and aims?

Is overall research methodology clearly identified and appropriate to research aims?

Are sufficient pre- and post- intervention data supplied for comparison groups?

Selection bias

How were participants allocated to groups?

How were confounding variables controlled for (eg matched by...)?

What variables were not controlled for (eg context, culture, setting)?

How was sample size controlled for?

Performance bias

Were recipients of intervention aware/unaware of assigned treatment?

Were other participants aware/unaware?

Is there any evidence of contamination, ie provision of intervention to control group?

Is there any evidence of context variables co-intervening, eg additional factors as possible influence?

Was exposure to intervention measured in a similar and unbiased way for both groups being compared?

Attrition bias

How was attrition managed?

Reporting bias

Were results reported for all predefined outcomes? (see Part 1)

Interpretations of findings from data

Are interpretations of results presented clearly with sufficient data analysis? (see Part 1)

Are interventions evaluated?

How adequate is the offered explanation to the problem, and to other research evidence?

Are alternative interpretations considered?

Are implications discussed in terms of:
a. addressing research aim?
b. suggesting further research?
c. impacting on policy/practice?
d. contribution to theory development/understanding in relation to other work?
e. by comparative methods for applicability to different populations/contexts/settings?

Are findings reliable and transferable?

Are findings useful for:
a. illuminating barriers?
b. identifying interventions?
c. evaluating of interventions?

Appendix 3:
Search strategies example:
PsychLIT

1. communication
2. barrier$
3. minority groups in DE
4. minority groups
5. ethnic groups in DE
6. ethnic
7. Asians in DE
8. race and ethnic discrimination in DE
9. multiculturalism in DE
10. 2 or 3 or 4 or 5 or 6 or 7 or 8 or 9
11. 1 and 10
12. health
13. communication skills in DE
14. communication skills training in DE
15. interpersonal communication in DE
16. verbal communication in DE
17. nonverbal communication in DE
18. 13 or 14 or 15 or 16 or 17
19. 12 and 18
20. cultural sensitivity in DE
21. evaluation in DE
22. intervention
23. or/20-22
24. 1 and 12 and 23
25. cross-cultural communication in DE
26. interpreters
27. (11 or 19 or 24 or 25 or 26) and (LA=English) and (PY=1989-2000)

Appendix 4: Tables

Interventions focused on linkworkers

Table 1: Comparison of interventions focused on linkworkers

Study Year	Mason 1990	Hoare et al 1994	Rocheron et al 1989
Aims	Assess the impact of linkworker intervention on Gujarati and Punjabi speaking Asian women's use and understanding of health care, and on health of babies.	Evaluate effectiveness of linkworker visits to Pakistani and Bangladeshi women's homes in increasing screening attendance.	Aims of evaluation – to give account of linkworker scheme with "Asian mothers" and identify key factors in its success or failure; to monitor any resultant changes in quality of care.
Methods	Comparative design involving linkworker intervention groups and control group. Questionnaire interviews on three occasions. Obstetric records collected.	Randomised controlled trial. Linkworkers trained to follow up intervention group a few weeks before screening interventions sent out. Attendance for screening recorded.	Multi-method study of three comparison districts over one year. Surveys and interviews with Asian mothers, midwives, managers, health visitors and linkworkers. Work records of linkworkers
Outcomes	Quantitative. Care and delivery measures; health outcome measures; health education measures; knowledge and use of service measures.	Measures of attendance at clinic for screening.	Some quantitative survey analysis of user and professional service satisfaction; qualitative analysis of observational and interview data on organisational practice, communication processes, and service use.
Findings	Small comparative increase for intervention group in health education knowledge and knowledge of available services, but no comparative increase in service use or health outcomes.	No significant overall difference in rates of attendance between control and intervention groups.	Impact of schemes influenced by lack of prior needs analysis or community involvement. Management, midwives and health visitors saw linkworker roles differently from linkworkers. Mothers' views were different again. Morale of linkworkers affected by terms of employment. Report claims linkworkers facilitated better communication and quality of care.

Interventions focused on interpreters

Table 2: Comparison of interventions focused on interpreters

Study Year	Baker, Parker et al 1996	Baker, Hayes et al 1998	Hornberger et al 1996
Aims	Assess how interpreter use affected Spanish-speaking patients' understanding of diagnosis and treatment plans.	Evaluate effects of interpreting practices on Spanish-speaking patients' satisfaction with interpersonal aspects of communication in interpreter-mediated examinations and examinations without interpreters at a public hospital emergency department.	Assess impact of two language interpretation services – including 'remote-simultaneous' service – on measures of interpreting quality and of clinician, interpreter and non-English-speaking patient satisfaction.
Methods	Spanish–peaking patients presenting to emergency department were interviewed prior to examination and, by telephone or face-to-face, one week after examination. Knowledge of diagnosis, treatment plans and follow-up appointments were assessed. Patients were asked whether they wanted interpreters and whether they used interpreters.	Spanish-speaking patients presenting to emergency department were interviewed prior to examination and, by telephone or face-to-face, one week after examination (same sample as Baker et al, 1996). Questionnaire was used to obtain satisfaction ratings for clinicians' communication. Patients were asked whether they wanted interpreters and whether they used interpreters.	Randomised controlled study comparing remote-simultaneous with proximate-consecutive services. Mothers alternated between two services at successive visits to 'well-baby clinic'. Interpreters had 15 hours of training in remote interpreting. Interactions audiotaped. Questionnaires for satisfaction ratings.
Outcomes	Patient self-reports on understanding of diagnosis, treatment, and appointments. Likert scale ratings of understandings. Hospital records used for comparison.	Five measures of interpersonal aspects of care used: friendliness; respect; concern; time spent; and making patient feel comfortable. Likert scale ratings.	Types and frequency of utterances by mother and physician. Accuracy of interpreter. Satisfaction ratings for mother, interpreter and physician.
Findings	Interpreters used were often untrained or were wanted and not provided. Use of interpreter gave better self-perceived understandings than when interpreter wanted but not used. But objective measures showed no difference. Best understandings for those who neither wanted nor used an interpreter.	Interpreters used were often untrained or were wanted and not provided. Having an 'ad hoc' interpreter was associated with less overall satisfaction with interpersonal aspects of care than not having one and not wanting one. But not having an interpreter when one was wanted gave worst satisfaction ratings.	Remote service resulted in more utterances by mother and physician and in greater accuracy of interpretation than proximate-consecutive interpretation. It was preferred by physicians and mothers but not by interpreters.

Interventions focused on communication training for health professionals

Table 3: Comparison of interventions focused on communication training

Study Year	Blackford 1996	Stolk et al 1998	Farnill et al 1997
Aims	Action research. First, nurses identify practice issues and recommend changes. Second, nurses implement changes. An emergent aim: increase usage of interpreter service.	Impact study to identify whether policy and training intervention would result in increase in number and length of interactions with patients in languages other than English.	Evaluate training intervention. Teaching interview skills to medical students, in order to enhance skills and increase sensitivity to multicultural issues.
Methods	Cycle: involving nurse planning, action, analysis, and reflection.	Non-comparative before- and-after study.	Non-comparative study of course using video and role-play. Skills ratings using volunteers, students, video raters.
Outcomes	Measures of interpreter use by nurses. Anecdotes.	Quantity and duration of interpreter bookings.	Skills items, eg listening and speaking. Ideas and feelings included.
Findings	Increase in interpreter use by nurses. Claims that nursing attitudes and practice improved, and interpreter service updated its profile.	Increase in length and duration of interpreter bookings sustained over six months. Bilingual staff contacts showed no significant increase.	Skills: volunteers, students and video raters rated course effective. Volunteers and video raters identified weakness in students' learning to show empathy.

Interventions focused on heart health education

Table 4: Comparison of interventions focused on heart health education

Study Year	Elder et al 1998	Brown et al 1996
Aims	Assess impact of nutrition education conducted in ESL classes on 'low literate Latino' students' nutrition-related knowledge, attitudes, behaviours, and physiological measures related to cardiovascular health.	Assess whether a heart health programme introducing Greek-Australian women to appropriate activities and encouraging them to reduce dietary fat intake would improve cardiovascular health.
Methods	Randomised parallel groups design. Intervention group given nutrition and heart health education integrated into ESL classes; control group at same college received stress management education. Physiological and psychological assessment measures collected at baseline, at three months and at six months. Data analysed to measure change across time and between comparison groups.	Comparison study of intervention group of women from Greek Orthodox Church community, and control group of women from neighbourhood community centre. Physiological and self-assessment data collected at pre-test, after 12 weeks of weekly meetings and home-based self-help sessions, and after 12 more weeks of home-based self-help sessions only. Data analysed to measure change across time and between comparison groups.
Outcomes	Measures of knowledge and attitudes – self-report; rating scale-based measures of nutrition-related psychosocial outcomes, eg fat avoidance; nutrition knowledge; intention to change; stress knowledge. Measures of physiological change, eg cholesterol measures, blood pressure.	Measures of physiological change, eg waist–hip ratios; blood pressure measures; exercise heart rates; self-reported dietary fat intake.
Findings	Intervention only had significant effects for fat avoidance and nutrition knowledge. But other variables showed no enduring group change.	Intervention had significant effects on body composition and aerobic fitness, whereas control group showed no change.

Interventions focused on use of health information materials with aim of increasing uptake of screening by minority ethnic users

Table 5: Comparison of interventions focused on use of health information materials with aim of increasing uptake of screening by minority ethnic users

Study Year	McAvoy and Raza 1991	Yancey et al 1995	Stone et al 1998
Aims	Assess effectiveness of using three types of material for home health education on the uptake of cervical screening by Asian women with several language backgrounds, in Leicester. The materials were video, leaflet, fact sheet. Assess, also, effectiveness of personal visits with materials compared with posted materials.	Evaluation of effectiveness of using 'culture-sensitive' videos placed in two community health clinic waiting rooms on the uptake of cervical screening among Latino women in New York and Los Angeles. The videos were in English and Spanish language formats.	Compare effectiveness on attendance of South Asian Gujarati speakers in Leicester for screening for infection with *Helicobacter pylori* (H pylori) of: a. sending screening invitations and information leaflets in English only; b. sending invitations in English with translated information leaflets and covering note in Gujarati.
Methods	Randomised controlled study. Two groups were visited personally and shown a video or a leaflet and fact sheet. One group was mailed a fact sheet and leaflet, one group received no contact.	Quasi-experimental study: one week 'on', one week 'off' design at the two sites. Videos were continuously displayed during 'on' weeks at each site to obtain the sample. 'Off' week samples served as controls. Follow-up data from monthly pap smears over three to five months.	Experimental study with randomised groups. At stage 1 Asian and non-Asian groups were invited to screen in English. At stage 2 a further matched group of Asians was selected from same sample frame and invited to screen with Gujarati material. Invitation letters sent through GPs stated screening was part of a research programme.
Outcomes	Attendance for smear testing measured within four months of intervention.	Monthly lab summary reports were compared with appointment records.	Reasons for non-attendance recorded from interviews with non-attenders. Attendances at screening sessions recorded.
Findings	The visited video method was most effective, followed by the visited leaflet and fact sheet method. Among the video group the best attendance results were for those viewing the video in own time, not with researcher.	Proportion of women who received pap smears was one third higher in video intervention group than in control group at each clinic.	Translated materials showed no gain over non-translated materials. Attendances low for all groups. There were few differences in attendance by ethnicity. The main reason given for non-attendance by Asians was 'too busy'.

Index

Page references for notes are followed by *n*

A

acculturation xxii
ad hoc interpreters 73, 83-7, 159
advocates xviii, 21, 158
  distribution of work 24
  intervention studies 51-5
  short-term funding 22
  training 23
affective empathy xxviii
Ahmad, W. v, xiv, xvii, xxi, 8, 9
Alleyne, J. xx
Annandale, E. xiii
Arai, Y. 19
Arora, R. viii, 2, 18, 20, 21, 22, 24, 25, 26
Asian Mother and Baby Campaign 56-61, 65-71
asylum seekers vi, 15, 16
Atkinson, P. xxvi
Atri, J. 93, 113-18, 122, 160
audio tapes 162
  intervention studies 138-42
audio-visual resources 26
  see also videotapes

B

Bahl, V. 23
Baker, D. 73, 79-87, 159, 196
Baker, E. 55
Bangladeshis, psychological distress 118-23
Barker, P. xxiii
barriers research x, 1-2
  presentation of findings xi-xii
  process barriers 3-14
  selection of studies x, 181-2
  structural barriers 15-30
  study protocol ix-x, 181
Baxter, C. 15, 16, 17, 21, 22, 23, 24
behavioural flexibility xxviii-xxix

Bhatt, A. 24, 25, 26
Bhatti-Sinclair, K. 33-7
biculturalism xxii
bilingual services xii, 1, 21-2, 30, 158-60
  employment profile mechanisms 23-4
  organisation 22-3
  service matching 41-9
  training 23
  see also advocates; interpreters; linkworkers
Bithell, C. 27
Blackford, J. 93-7, 107, 112, 113, 123, 160, 197
Bowes, A. 8, 14
Bowler, I.M.W. 7
Box, V. 26
breast screening 61-4, 113-18
Brown, P. 12
Brown, W. 125, 130-4, 163, 198
Buckinghamshire Health Authority 16

C

cardiovascular disease, health education 125-30, 198
caring models, adaptation 3-6
cervical smear testing 142-51
Chahal, K. 23
child development 138-42
Chow, P. 17
Chu, C. xix
Clevely Northgate Trust 16
Clinical governance (DoH) vi, 1, 162
cognitive flexibility xxviii
Commission for Racial Equality (CRE) xvi
  Race Relations Code of Practice in Primary Health Care 34

communication
　and culture xxiii–xxix
　and ethnicity xiv–xv
　and racism xvii, xix
communication barriers 1–2
　process barriers 3–14
　structural 15–30
communication needs xi, xviii,
　15–18, 29, 157, 165
community project workers
　(CPWs) 118–23
complaints procedures 18
confidentiality xxvii, 13, 20–1
consultation xi, xviii, 16
Crystal, D. xxx *n*
Culley, L. xix
cultural communicative competence
　xxviii
cultural difference xix–xxi
　and miscommunication xxiv
culture xiii
　allowing for diversity xxi–xxiii
　and communication xxiii–xxix
　cultural difference and health
　　beliefs xix–xxi
　and gender 8–10
　and language 10–13

D

data extraction form xi, 183, 185–92
Davis, S. vii, 20, 21, 38–41, 157
Day, S. 51–5, 56, 61, 158
Department of Health (DoH) 166
　organisational reforms 15
　policy documents vi, 1, 162
diabetes, health education 135–8
Dickinson, R. 24, 25, 26
disabled vi
diversity xxi–xxiii
divided attention xxvii
Domokos, T. 8, 14
Dowoo, P. 26–7
dynamism xxi–xxiii

E

Ehlers, M. 26–7
Elder, J. 125–9, 134, 198

emergency departments 79–87
empathy 13
empirical barrier studies *see* barriers
　research
empowerment 15
ethnic matching xii, 41–9
ethnic minority xxx *n*
ethnic monitoring xii, 1, 20–1, 157
　intervention studies 38–41
ethnicity
　and communication xiv–xv
　definitions xiii
　and health xiii–xiv
external audit 33–7

F

family members, as interpreters 13
Farnill, D. 93, 97–103, 112, 113, 117,
　160, 197
Farooq, S. xxvi, 13, 87–90
Farrow, S. 19
Farshi, Z. 1, 19, 21, 93, 103–8, 122,
　161
Fenton, S. 11
flashcards 135–8
fluency v, xxx *n*
Free, C. 15, 17

G

gender xxiii
　and culture 8–10
Gerrish, K. viii, xxviii, 1, 3, 4, 13, 23,
　27, 28–9
Gillam, S. 21, 22, 23
Good, B. xxvi
Good, M. xxvi
Goodman, M. 21
GPs *see* primary care
Greek migrants, heart health
　program 130–4
Green, J. 1, 21
Greenwood, J. 14, 162
Guarnaccia, P. xxi, xxii
Gudykunst, W. xxviii
Gumperz, J. xxiv

H

Hall, J. xxv
Hasselkus, B. 13
Hatton, C. 24
Hatton, D. 13
Hawthorne, K. 102, 134, 135–8, 164
health advocates *see* advocates
health care professionals, attitudes
    and practices vii, viii
health education xii, 163–6
    intervention studies 125–38, 142–
    51, 198, 199
health research
    ethnicity xiii–xiv
    racism xvii–xix
heart, health education 125–34, 198
Hedges, C. 93, 118–23, 161
Helicobacter pylori 151–6
Heritage, J. xxvi
Hoare, T. 56, 61–4, 70, 146, 158, 195
holistic care 3–5
Holland, J. xx
Hornberger, J. xxvi, 13, 73, 74–9, 83,
    87, 159, 196
Hyden, L–C. xxv, xxvi

I

Ilett, S. 134, 138–42
indirect racism xvi–xvii
institutional racism vii–viii,
    xvi–xvii, 7, 14
intercultural communicative
    competence xxviii
interpreters xii, xviii, 73, 159–60,
    196
    distribution of work 24
    emergency departments 79–87
    primary care xxvii, 21
    psychiatry 87–91, 108–13
    remote-simultaneous
        interpretation 74–9
    training 103–8, 161
intervention studies x, 31–2
    advocates and linkworkers 51–71
    conclusions 157–66
    data extraction form xi, 183,
        185–92

health education programmes and
    resources 125–56, 198, 199
    interpreters 73–91, 196
    linkworkers 55–71, 137–8, 195
    practitioner training 93–123, 197
    presentation of findings xii
    selection x, 181–2
    service development 33–49
    study protocol ix–x, 181
    isolation 5

J

Jaggi, A. 27
Johnson, K. xxx *n*
Johnson, M. vii

K

Kai, J. 93, 118–23, 161
Karim, J. viii, 9, 16, 17, 18, 20, 21,
    22, 25, 26
Kelleher, D. xxi, xxiii
Kim, Y. xxviii
King, F. xv

L

Lam, T. 1, 21
Lambert, H. xix, xxi
language xi
    and ethnicity xiii
    process barriers 10–13
Language Line 79
language matching 41–9
Law, I. xiii, xvi
Lawrenson, R. 1, 18, 20, 21
Leather, C. 21, 23
Leeds NHS Interpreting Project
    103–8
Leets, L. xiv, xv
Leininger, M. xx
Lemmer, B. xi
Levenson, R. 21, 22, 23
Levinson, S. 12
linkworkers xviii, 16, 21, 158–9
    distribution of work 24
    intervention studies 55–71, 137–8,
        195

management structure 22
short-term funding 22
training 23
literature search x-xi, 183, 193
Lupton, D. xxvi, xxvii

M

McAvoy, B. 8, 65, 117, 138, 142-7, 150, 151, 156, 164, 199
Macleod Clark, J. viii, 4, 5
McNamara, B. 1, 27
MacPherson Report vii, xvi, 7
McTear, M. xv
Making a difference (Doh) vi, 1
management structure, bilingual services 22-3
marking race xvi
Martin, J. xxiii, xxiv
Mason, E. 56-61, 64, 70, 158, 195
material resources vii, viii, xii, xviii, 164
  intervention studies 134-56
  quality 26
  translation 25
  variety 26-7
Maynard, D. xxvi
Mays, N. xi
meanings 10-11
  in context 11-12
medical students 97-103
men vi, 8
methodology
  advisory panel ix
  data extraction form xi, 183, 185-92
  intervention studies 31
  search strategy x, 183, 193
  selection of studies x, 181-2
  study protocol ix-x, 181
Miles, R. xvi
mindfulness xxviii, xxix
minority ethnic v, xxix n
minority ethnic practitioners 29
miscommunication xi, xv, xviii, 30, 157
  and culture xxiv
  process barriers 10-13

Mishler, E. xxv, xxvi
Mitchell, P. 22
Monach, J. vii, 20, 21, 38-41, 157
monitoring *see* ethnic monitoring
Multi-Ethnic Women's Health Project (MEWHP) 52
multi-party communication 12-13, 162
Murphy, K. viii, 4, 5

N

Naish, J. 19
Nakayama, T. xxiii, xxiv
Nazroo, J. xiii, xiv
negative attribution xvi
Newman, M. xi
nurses
  caring models 3-6
  interpreter use 93-7

O

older people vi, 25, 26
organisational barriers *see* structural barriers
over-controlling behaviour viii

P

Pakistanis
  flashcard health education 135-8
  psychological distress 118-23
pap smears 142-51
Papadopoulos, I. xx, xxviii, 3
Parsons, L. 51-5, 56, 61, 158
Pauwels, A. xx-xxi, 6-7, 10-12, 13
Phipps, D. 6
pictorial materials 26-7, 135-8, 164
Piracha, A. 9, 15
Plunkett, A. 24
Podro, S. 23
Popay, J. xi
Pope, C. xi
power differences xxvii
practitioner education *see* training
primary care
  ethnic and language monitoring 21, 38-41

gender issues 8-9
interpreters 21
structural barriers 19
process barriers
adaptation of prevailing models 3-6
culture, gender and communication styles 8-10
implications for practitioners 13-14
language, culture and miscommunication 10-13
stereotyping 6-7
professional training *see* training
psychiatry, interpreters 87-90, 108-13
psychological distress 118-23

Q

qualitative research xi
quantitative research xi
Quine, S. 24

R

Race Relations (Amendment) Act 2000 vii, xv, xvii, 7
racialisation xiv, xvii
racism xv-xvii
bilingual services 23
and health xvii-xix
institutional vii-viii, 14
Raza, R. 8, 15, 65, 117, 138, 142-7, 150, 151, 164, 199
receptionists 19-20, 160-1
training 113-18
records, patient access 18
referrals 2, 21
reflective ability xxviii-xxix
refugees 15, 16
Rehbein, J. 13
remote-simultaneous interpretation 74-9
residential care 24
resource allocation, principles 6, 17
review findings, presentation xi-xii
Ritch, A. 6, 17

Roberts, C. xxiv, 12
Robinson, L. v, xxi
Rocheron, Y. viii, 22, 23, 56, 65-71, 146, 159, 195
Rodriguez, O. xxi, xxii
Rodwell, C. 3
Roter, D. xxv

S

Sadiq Sangster, A. 11
Saldov, M. 17
Sarangi, S. xxiv
Saving lives (DoH) vi, 1, 162
Scollon, R. xxiv
Scollon, S. xxiv
screening 199
breast cancer 61-4, 113-18
cervical smear testing 142-51
Helicobacter pylori 151-6
Sefi, S. xxvi
self-management 15
service matching xii, 41-9
service provision xii, 17, 163
external audit 33-7
Shah, R. 9, 14, 15, 26
Shea, A. 16, 22, 26
Silove, D. 42-6, 158
Silverman, D. xviii, xxvi
situational ethnicity xiii
Sivak, L. xix, xxi
Smaje, C. xiii, xviii
Small, R. 18, 28
Snowden, L. 46-9, 158
Sourial, S. 3
South Asians vi, 1, 7
speaking-about-patients model xxvi, xxvii
speaking-by-patients model xxvi, xxvii
speaking-to-patients model xxv
speaking-with-patients model xxv -xxvi, xxvii
Stephenson, P. 15
stereotyping viii, xi, xviii, xx-xxi, 14, 157
Stolk, Y. 93, 107, 108-13, 117, 122, 160, 197

Stone, M. 117, 142, 146, 151-6, 199
structural barriers 1, 15, 29-30
  bilingual services 21-4
  getting through the system 18-21
  implications for health
    practitioners 29
  material resources and media 25-7
  professional training and
    communication practice 27-9
  user need and access 15-18
study protocol ix-x, 181

T

Tomlinson, S. 102, 134, 135-8, 164
training xii, 30, 160-3, 197
  bilingual health workers 23
  clinical psychiatric staff 108-13
  interpreters 103-8, 161
  local residents 118-23
  medical students 97-103
  nurses 93-7
  process barriers 13-14
  receptionists 113-18
  structural barriers 27-9
transcultural communication
    competence 162, 165
  models xi, xxiii, xxv-xxix
translation xxvi, 13, 25
Trill, M. xx
Trinh, Q. 15, 16
trust 20

U

user communication needs xi, xviii,
    15-18, 29, 157, 165
user involvement, research 118-23,
    161

V

videotapes 162
  health education 26, 142-51, 164
  for training 97-103
Vietnamese 42-6
Vital connection, The (DoH) vi, 21
Vydelingum, V. 1, 5

W

Warrier, S. 21
Webb, T. 13
Wheal, A. 33-7
women, process barriers 8-10, 14

Y

Yancey, A. 138, 142, 146, 147-51,
    156, 164, 199